CANCER MANAGEMENT WITH CHINESE MEDICINE

CANCER MANAGEMENT

WITH CHINESE MEDICINE

YU RENCUN
Beijing Hospital of Traditional Chinese Medicine, China

HONG HAI
Nanyang Technological University, Singapore

World Scientific

NEW JERSEY · LONDON · SINGAPORE · BEIJING · SHANGHAI · HONG KONG · TAIPEI · CHENNAI

Published by

World Scientific Publishing Co. Pte. Ltd.

5 Toh Tuck Link, Singapore 596224

USA office: 27 Warren Street, Suite 401-402, Hackensack, NJ 07601

UK office: 57 Shelton Street, Covent Garden, London WC2H 9HE

British Library Cataloguing-in-Publication Data
A catalogue record for this book is available from the British Library.

ISBN-13 978-981-4374-74-3
ISBN-10 981-4374-74-1

Typeset by Stallion Press
Email: enquiries@stallionpress.com

Printed in Singapore.

CONTENTS

---

* Translated and edited by Hong Hai

ABOUT THE AUTHORS

Yu Rencun is Honorary Director and Professor at the Beijing Hospital of Traditional Chinese Medicine. He was trained in Western medicine before undergoing an extensive course in Traditional Chinese Medicine (TCM). He has been engaged in cancer research for over 50 years and treated numerous cancer patients in China and various parts of Southeast Asia. He has been Advisor to the Oncology Committee of the Chinese Association for the Integration of Traditional and Western Medicine and the Singapore Thong Chai Medical Institution. For his outstanding contributions to cancer treatment and TCM, Professor Yu has been awarded over 20 prizes by the China Ministry of Health and the Beijing Municipal Government.

Hong Hai is Professorial Fellow at the Nanyang Technological University (NTU) and Senior Fellow at NTU's Institute of Advanced Studies. Trained originally in engineering and economics, Professor Hong later studied Chinese medicine and qualified as a registered TCM physician in Singapore and researched the scientific basis for TCM for his doctoral dissertation at the Beijing University of Chinese Medicine. He has previously served on the Singapore TCM Practitioners Board and practises at the Public Free Clinic and the Renhai Clinic.

PREFACE

Traditional Chinese Medicine (TCM) as a system of healing and health preservation has much to offer in the prevention and management of cancers. For patients who have contracted the ailment, TCM is generally not able to offer a complete cure although there have been claims and anecdotal evidence relating to successful treatments.

Playing a complementary role to Western medical treatments of cancer is where TCM can make, and has made, important contributions. Cancer patients usually exhibit clinical conditions that TCM recognize as internal disorders, such as poor flow of qi, blood stasis, deficiency of qi or blood, and internal heat. Treatments like surgery, chemotherapy and radiotherapy often leave the patient with severe side effects and in a weakened state. TCM treatments can help the patient manage these conditions by strengthening the immune system, facilitating flow, and eliminating toxins. This helps the patient in recovery or brings about a better quality of life.

This book offers the reader the benefit of Professor Yu's decades of experience combining TCM therapy with Western treatments of cancer. It also provides advice on diet and living habits that help prevent cancer or assist in recovery.

For those unfamiliar with TCM theory, we have included intro-
ductory chapters on TCM principles and herbal medications.

We gratefully acknowledge the assistance of Dr Zhang
Zhichen of the Beijing University of Chinese Medicine and
TCM physicians Karen Wee and Doreen Low of Nanyang
Technological University in the translation to English of parts
of book.

CHAPTER 1

INTRODUCTION

Cancer is a complex family of diseases. In recent decades, rapid advances in the introduction of new drugs, surgical interventions and other therapeutic methods have been made by modern medicine in the treatment of cancers. Many early-stage cancers can now be cured and life can be prolonged for late-stage cancers with these new methods.

Traditional Chinese Medicine (TCM) does not in general offer treatment of cancers with a view to the complete elimination of disease. Rather, it directs itself to helping the body to strengthen and balance itself to give the patient the best chance of overcoming or living with the disease. After patients have undergone chemotherapy, radiotherapy and/or surgery, TCM can often help fortify the patient against the side effects of these therapies, or repair the immune system that has been affected by the toxicity of certain drugs used in chemotherapy. In some instances, with the consent of the Western oncologist treating the patient, TCM herbs can be used concurrently with chemotherapy and radiotherapy to help the patient cope with the side effects of those treatments.

Professor Yu Rencun was trained in Western medicine with specialization in oncology. Through his study of Chinese medicine and his clinical work, mostly at the Beijing Hospital of

Traditional Chinese Medicine where Western and Chinese methods are used together for a whole range of illnesses, he has gathered a wealth of experience using Chinese herbal medicine as a complementary treatment for patients who have undergone Western medical therapies.

In recent years he has spent a considerable amount of time treating patients in various parts of Asia, in particular Singapore which he visits regularly as a clinical consultant. He has written over 20 books on cancer and related subjects. This book, the first of his works to be written in English, captures the essence of the methods that he has used and documents a number of typical cases in which herbal medicine is used to manage cancer patients to improve their quality of life and, in some instances, to prolong their lives.

It is my privilege to have been acquainted with Professor Yu for over 20 years and observed many of the cases satisfactorily treated by him. I was therefore pleased that he asked me to collaborate with him in writing this book in English in order that his vast experience and deep insights into the role that TCM can play in cancer management be recorded for an English-speaking audience. This audience would include not only medical professionals but also patients and their relatives who can benefit from better understanding the conditions of the patients and appreciating how TCM could help in the management of these conditions.

The book would also be useful to the general reader who wishes to know how TCM works and how it can be applied to cultivating health and keeping his body in good condition to prevent this and other similar diseases.

Chapter 2 gives an outline of the concepts and principles in TCM. This is essential reading for those who are not trained in TCM or familiar with its main body of theory. The next chapter introduces the reader to Chinese herbs and how they are combined for therapeutic and health promotion purposes.

Chapter 4 describes how TCM looks at cancer as a disease and the principles employed in therapy. It draws heavily on Professor Yu's scholarly writings. As it attempts to present the subject in a manner to which a Western-educated readership can more easily relate, this and subsequent chapters do not attempt a literal translation of any part or parts of Professor Yu's earlier works, and may not always conform to the standard terminology used in English translations of TCM textbooks. (It should be noted, though, that there is as yet no universally accepted standard terminology for translating TCM, this being a subject of continuing discussion and debate in academic and regulatory circles.)

Where I have occasionally taken the liberty to use more appropriate terms to help the reader understand the concepts, I make no apologies for doing so as our aim is to help the reader gain an understanding of the ideas and principles involved rather than to provide a reference text for medical professionals and students. For example, "dysphoria" is the technical term used to translate "*xinfan*" (心烦), "a sensation of stuffiness with heat in the chest and irritableness"[1] sometimes associated with stagnation of liver *qi*. I have in some contexts used the term "irritability" to translate "*xinfan*".

Chapter 5 deals with five major categories of cancer to illustrate the principles and methods employed and the results achieved. These cases are drawn from Professor Yu's medical files from the 1970s to 2006. These cases are but a few of a more comprehensive list cited in an earlier publication in Chinese.[2]

---

1 *Chinese-English Dictionary of Traditional Chinese Medicine.* (1996) Renmin Weisheng Publishing House, Beijing, p. 229.

2 Yu Rencun *et al.* (ed.) (2007) *Yu Rencun* 郁仁存, China Press of Traditional Chinese Medicine, Beijing.

The final chapter deals with the prevention of cancer and the management of diets and daily living habits for cancer patients. This is a useful chapter for the general reader who wishes to understand Chinese medicine for health cultivation and disease prevention. Chapters 2, 3 and 6 in combination can therefore be read in isolation from the rest of the book as a general introduction to TCM, health cultivation and the prevention of cancer.

The TCM Approach to Cancer Management

The TCM management of cancer described in this book is holistic in the sense that, unlike Western medicine, it does not focus on the destruction or containment of cancer cells. It looks at the presence of a malignant tumour as the result of imbalances in the body's internal host environment that leads to abnormal cell growth. Its approach to management of the disease is therefore one of creating and regulating this internal environment to give the patient's own body the best chance of defending itself and/or co-existing with the cancer cells.

TCM oncologists like Professor Yu recognize and understand the power of Western drugs, radiotherapy and surgery in removing, destroying and containing tumours and cancer cells. They also believe in the judicious integration of Western and Chinese healing methods to give the patient the best of both worlds: one treats the disease; the other strengthens the host body to do battle with the disease by resolving internal imbalances known as TCM syndromes. If one may be allowed to use a somewhat invidious analogy, Western methods can be compared to the use of overwhelming force to attack the military bases of an occupying enemy, with accompanying collateral damage, destroying the homes and lives of innocent civilians. Chinese medical therapy, on the other hand, would be the equivalent of soft power used to build up the resistance of local people to repel and contain foreign enemy forces. Working together, they can achieve a much better result than would be possible with each acting alone. The selected cases presented here from Professor Yu's medical files will help illustrate this principle.

Hong Hai
December 2011

CHAPTER 2

PRINCIPLES OF DIAGNOSIS AND THERAPY IN TRADITIONAL CHINESE MEDICINE

Chinese medicine as practised today in China, some East Asian countries and the West is both an art and a science. To the extent that it has a scientific aspect to it, we can regard it as an empirically based form of healing that has progressed over the centuries by drawing on the accumulated clinical experience of successful physicians as well as — albeit to a lesser extent — modern scientific knowledge of anatomy and physiology.

Ancient Chinese medicine was formalized as a system of thought and practice after the founding of the People's Republic of China in 1949. "Traditional Chinese medicine" (TCM) is the common term for the modernized form of Chinese medicine.

TCM is described as "traditional" to indicate that it is derived from ancient medicine. It retains many of the core concepts and theories of ancient medicine and is based on a body of theory distinct from that of Western medicine practised in Chinese hospitals and clinics today. TCM is taught through medical degree courses in Chinese universities as well as tertiary institutions in East Asia, Australia, Europe and North America. In most of these countries, these courses are prerequisites for registration as licensed TCM practitioners by health authorities. Although Western medicine is dominant and is the mainstream form of medicine practised in these countries, TCM plays a significant and recognized role in national healthcare in China (including Hong Kong and Taiwan), Japan, Korea, Malaysia and Singapore, and has a sizeable and growing following in many Western countries.[1]

TCM should also be distinguished from Chinese folk medicine handed down largely by word of mouth and practised unregulated (strictly speaking, illegitimately) in China and some other Asian countries. Such folk medicine may have arcane practices like blood-letting, divination and the use of unusual drugs and animal parts not listed in the Chinese pharmacopoeia. The concepts and principles discussed in this book are not concerned with Chinese folk medicine.

It should be noted that the selective use of *materia medica* (herbs) and herbal formulations by Western doctors as complementary treatments for disease is not part of TCM. By way of analogy, when Western doctors use quinine for the treatment of malaria they are not practising Indian medicine, even though the drug was originally extracted from a South American tree used by native Indians to treat fever. Likewise, extracts of the ginkgo leaf used by German scientists to manufacture ginkgo biloba, which is claimed to promote blood circulation, is not Chinese medicine, even though the ginkgo nut is a common ingredient of standard Chinese medications. Most clinical trials on Chinese herbs have been done with a view to discovering new drugs for Western medicine. The use of such drugs and information

---

[1] Korean medicine is practised as a slight variation of TCM. Many Korean physicians receive postgraduate training at Chinese universities.

derived from clinical trials do not directly pertain to the theory and treatment methodologies of TCM, although they may contain useful information for the latter. For the same reason, the selective borrowing of acupuncture techniques by Western doctors to relieve pain does not amount to the practice of TCM.

To understand TCM better, it is useful to review briefly its history. For readers who want to skip this, please go directly to Section 2.3.

2.1. Origins of Chinese Medical Theory

Many of the concepts in TCM today can be found in ancient cosmology and metaphysics. The basic theory of ancient Chinese medicine was derived partly from ancient cosmological models, albeit modified and reinterpreted over many centuries in the light of empirical experience. The literature of the history of medicine in China provides insights into how Chinese medical thought has evolved from ancient times and holds useful clues to understanding the epistemology of its theory.

Ancient Chinese medicine, like the ancient Greco-Roman medicine of Hippocrates and Galen, dates back several thousand years. The concepts of *yin* and *yang*, which are central to Chinese medical theory, go back to the *I-Ching* (*The Book of Changes*) written early in the Zhou dynasty (1046–256 BC) and to Taoism whose founder was Lao Tzu (circa 600 BC). The concept of *qi* (气) appeared originally in ancient Chinese cosmology as a formless substance that pervaded the universe at the beginning of time. *Qi* materialized into all the elements that made up the cosmos and also was the source of all energy and change. This pervasive and ubiquitous nature of *qi* later found its way into medicine. However, within the medical literature, it had a more restricted meaning, though still wide enough that one scholar has estimated that in the medical classic *Huangdi neijing* alone there are some 1700 mentions of *qi* with varying shades of meaning.[2]

Other entities like *jing* 精 (essence), wind, dampness and heat similarly have multiple meanings depending on the context. They are therefore troublesome to grapple with for a Western medical scientist trying to understand the theory and concepts of TCM.

The first comprehensive manual of Chinese medical theory was the *Huangdi Neijing* (*The Inner Canon of the Yellow Emperor*) compiled by various authors during the Han dynasty (206 BC to AD 220). The *Neijing* was arguably the first medical manual that treated medicine as an empirical science. Before the *Neijing*, Chinese medicine was dominated by the belief that illness was caused by spirits and demons and required the intervention of witches and mediums to effect cures. Ancient Greek and Roman temple medicine was also dominated by similar beliefs, treating the sick by having mythological gods intervene in their dreams. The *Neijing* made a break with this tradition by refusing to attribute disease causation to numinous agents, focusing instead on environmental conditions and emotional factors as the causes of illness and on natural laws in their explanation.[3] It established the idea of systematic correspondence by which all tangible and abstract phenomena could be categorized as manifestations of certain cosmological models, the main ones being the *yin-yang* principle and the five-phase model.

The *Neijing's* principal breakthrough insight was to base medicine on common sense and empirical observation. It postulates that there is a normal healthy state of the body that

---

[2] Wang (2001), p. 44.
[3] Unschuld (2003), p. 319.

manifests in observable signs in a healthy person — the complexion of his face, the spirited look in his eyes, the colour of his tongue and the kind of fur (coating) that sits on it, the tone and strength of his pulse, his bowel movements, his appetite, sleep habits, tolerance of heat and cold, and so on. Deviations from this normal healthy state point to imbalances in the body, and the role of the physician is to identify the nature of these imbalances and apply therapeutic techniques to rebalance the body. When imbalance occurs, herbs and acupuncture are used in accordance with the basic principles of *yin-yang* and the five elements to nudge the body in the direction of balance. In effect, Chinese therapeutic methods aim fundamentally to help the body heal itself.

Different schools of thought built around the basic tenets of the *Neijing* flourished from the Han dynasty to modern times, but they shared the core concepts and principles contained in the *Neijing*. *The Treatise on Febrile Diseases* (*Shanghan Lun* 伤寒论) by the legendary late-Han physician Zhang Zhongjing (150–219) postulated that harm caused by climatic influences such as cold and dampness travelled along (acupuncture) meridians and brought about progressive stages of pathogenesis. The Song dynasty (960–1279) saw the emergence of Neo-Confucianism, which in turn stimulated the development of new medical doctrines. The late Song and the ensuing Jin-Yuan dynasties saw vigorous contention among "a hundred schools" of medical thought. Among the influential schools were the Cold Damage School (*hanliang pai* 寒凉派), founded by *Liu Wansu* (1120–1200), which stressed cooling the body to overcome the tendency towards excess heat; the Stomach-Spleen School (*piwei pai* 脾胃派) of Li Dongyuan (1180–1251), who regarded the digestive system as the fundamental basis for good health; and the *Yin*-Nourishing School (*ziyin pai* 滋阴派) of Zhu Danxi (1281–1358), who emphasized nourishing the *yin* of the body as the basis for good health. The late Ming and early Qing saw further development of medical thought, notably studies of infectious diseases common in spring and summer in the south by the Warm Disorders School (*wenbing xuepai* 温病学派) led by Wu Youxing (1582–1652).

Although these contending schools were fundamentally based on the *Neijing*, they were also in tune with their times and the climate and social condition of the regions in which they flourished. For example, the Stomach-Spleen School was developed in the declining years of the Song dynasty when times were uncertain and people's lives were filled with sustained anxiety (*si* 思). Such anxiety, in TCM theory, leads to damage of the functions of the spleen and stomach. Likewise, during the era of Zhu Danxi, many wealthy merchants and members of the aristocracy often ate rich food excessively. Many led dissolute lives of indulgence in wine and women, leading to injury of the *yin* of the kidney and liver. The correct therapeutic approach then was to nourish the *yin* (滋阴).

2.2. The Establishment of Traditional Chinese Medicine

In the final decades of the Qing dynasty (1644–1911), foreign powers annexed territories and extracted war indemnities. Following the founding of the Chinese Republic in 1912, the May 4th Movement of 1919 marked a historic turning point when the country adopted Western science and technology as the only practical way of strengthening itself.[4] From the 1920s, as young scholars returned from studies abroad with the mission to modernize science in China, Chinese medicine came under attack for being unscientific. In 1929 a Japanese-educated Western doctor

---

[4] Schwartz (1986).

Yu Yan in the government health administration called for the abolition of Chinese medicine. This met with a robust response from Chinese physician and scholar Yun Tieqiao.[5] In the ensuing national debate, Western-trained scientists followed a line of thinking inspired by logical positivists whose ideas were gaining currency in Europe. They deemed unobservables like *qi* in Chinese medicine as metaphysical, hence meaningless, and Chinese medical theory to be unverifiable (or unfalsifiable), hence unscientific. Logical positivism has since gone out of fashion among philosophers of science, but its influence on the thinking of scientists continued for generations of scientists. Even today, one often comes across young scientists and doctors who believe only in the existence of what can be observed directly or through scientific instruments, and only in theories that can be expressed directly or indirectly by mathematical formulations.

Chinese physicians defended their profession by citing its successful clinical record and by appealing to the wisdom of ancient Chinese philosophy that explained medical theory. The first defence was difficult for Western doctors to deny, as there was a great deal of *prima facie* evidence for the efficacy of many Chinese medications and of acupuncture. Instead they insisted that this evidence be further subjected to rigorous clinical trials. However, the second defence, invoking the wisdom of an ancient philosophical system, convinced few detractors.

The debate was interrupted by civil war (1935–1949) that culminated in the ascendancy of Mao and the founding of the People's Republic of China in 1949. Early in his rule, Mao, a self-styled philosopher-king who believed deeply in ancient wisdom while recognizing the power of Western technology, directed that

---

[5] Ou (2005) and Lei (1999).

the country preserve the "treasure trove" of Chinese medicine and modernize it by absorbing relevant knowledge from Western science and medicine.[6]

Paradoxically, this modernized, state-sanctioned form of Chinese medicine henceforth became known as traditional Chinese medicine. Traditional only in sharing common concepts and models with the ancient Chinese medical classics, it was in fact viewed as a reformed system that reflected the social and political milieu of modern China.[7] Following Mao's edict to modernize TCM, textbooks were written in plain Chinese prose (*baihua*) as distinct from terse formal classical Chinese, systematically laying out the principles of TCM for the training of a new generation of Chinese doctors. This was in contrast to the old way of medical apprentices memorizing the classics and learning practice at the feet of experienced practitioners. The new texts were written by hand-picked leading scholars, mostly from new TCM colleges set up in Beijing, Chengdu, Guangzhou, Nanjing and Shanghai.

The first national TCM textbook appeared in 1958, titled *Outline of Chinese Medicine* (*Zhongyixue gailun* 中医学概论).[8] It was superseded by other specialized texts covering foundational theory, diagnostics, acupuncture and moxibustion, *materia medica*, prescriptions, internal medicine, paediatrics, gynaecology, skin diseases and so forth. The structural similarity of these textbooks to their Western medical counterparts was obvious and deliberate. The textbooks constituted a massive systematization of medical theory and practice, the first to take place in Chinese history.

---

[6] Taylor (2005).

[7] Farquhar (1994) and Scheid (2002).

[8] The 1972 text *A Revised Outline of Chinese Medicine* (新编中医学概要) was translated by Sivin (1987).

Regulation of TCM practice is by licensing of medical practitioners at the state level with common national examinations. Prescribed textbooks currently comprise a series published by Shanghai Science and Technology Press, which have also been adopted in Hong Kong and Singapore. Chinese medicine as practised in Taiwan and Malaysia follows a similar pattern, as does Korean medicine, which is basically an indigenized version of Chinese medicine.

TCM colleges in China require about 40% of the student's time to be spent on studying Western medicine. Graduates can practise basic Western medicine in addition to TCM. They are trained to read modern diagnostic test results, prescribe Western drugs and perform simple surgical procedures. Postgraduate students and researchers in Chinese medical colleges publish extensively in academic journals. While the rigour of research has yet to catch up with that of leading Western academic institutions, the existence of these postgraduate research programmes and publications indicate a decisive shift away from the unconditional acceptance of ancient philosophy to evidence-based medicine.

As Sivin notes, these changes were due to "unmistakable influence from modern medicine," whilst Scheid observes that the transition was not without its controversies and contends that despite the apparent uniformity forced upon the TCM community by state-sanctioned textbooks and clinical practices, there remains a plurality of views among scholars and practitioners.[9] Scheid's observation is especially pertinent considering influential conservative scholars like Liu Lihong who, despite having undergone training in systematized TCM, regard the ancient classics as the source of ultimate authority in medicine, and view modern

---

[9] Sivin (1987), p. 124; and Scheid (2002).

systematized TCM as Chinese medicine adulterated and distorted by Western influence.

The core principle of syndrome differentiation (see Section 2.4.3) and choosing the appropriate therapeutic method accordingly (*bianzheng lunzhi* 辨证论治) was given formal emphasis and became the core of Chinese medical practice.[10] TCM distinguished itself from Western medicine, with its emphasis on diseases and their causes, by focusing on *syndromes* (*zheng* 证) based on imbalances in the body and on methods of resolving them to restore health. (TCM syndromes and the principal TCM models are discussed further along in this chapter.)

2.3. Core Concepts and Entities in TCM

The core theory and concepts in TCM were developed at a time when very little was understood about human anatomy and physiology. Unlike Greece and Rome in antiquity, ancient China forbade dissections because the human body was considered sacred. Ancient Chinese descriptions of the human body organs and substances contained therein were therefore extremely simple and conjectural and the theory built on these entities and their functions was likewise highly simplistic compared to those of modern physiology and pathology. Yet a system of medicine was developed that provided the mainstay of healing for thousands of years, and was only partially supplanted by Western medicine as mainstream medicine in China in the middle of the 20th century.

As most TCM entities are unobservable and the theory based on them largely untested by clinical trials, the familiar epistemological questions in the philosophy of science naturally arise: Do

---

[10] Scheid (2002), pp. 106–115.

they really exist as we imagine them to be? What is the validity of theory based upon such entities and forming the basis of a healing system that has endured in scientifically developed societies like China, Japan and Korea?

The ancient Chinese picture of the human body is well documented in textbooks in Chinese as well as Western commentary.[11] It is important to understand from the outset that this picture is an abstraction of anatomical and physiological realities, that although terms like "blood" and "liver" are used to refer to what resemble the same entities in modern medicine, they in fact amounted to an attempt to incorporate all the essential functions of the body within a simple framework of a few fluids, organs and communication channels (meridians). By giving multiple complex functions to these basic entities, Chinese medicine built up models for the diagnosis and treatment of illnesses that appear to have served well as a system of healing from ancient times, although by modern standards it is clearly inadequate and can at best serve only as alternative or complementary medicine to modern Western medicine. With these limitations in mind, let us take a brief look at the simplified picture of the human body provided by TCM.

In the TCM model the human body comprises the following:

- *qi* (气), blood (*xue* 血) and clear body fluids (*jinye* 津液);
- meridians (channels) and branches (collaterals) (*jingluo* 经络) that serve as transport channels for *qi* and are connected to the organs;

---

[11] Among Western works, Kuriyama's much-cited *The Expressiveness of the Body* (1999) provides a largely historical account of the Chinese picture of the human body, with valuable insights into the evolution of key concepts and comparisons with pictures of the human body in Greco-Roman antiquity.

- solid (*zang*) and hollow (*fu*) organs (脏腑);
- the brain and marrow; the uterus (for females);
- muscles, skin and bones;
- the mind (*shen* 神), which has a close relationship with the body.

Different emotions are associated with the mind, each of which has a specific relationship to a particular organ (see a later section in this chapter).

2.3.1. The body's three essential substances: *qi*, blood and *jinye*

2.3.1.1. *Qi*

"*Qi*" is a word that is used extensively in the Chinese language, and can be used to refer to the profound and mysterious substance that pervaded the universe at the beginning of time in Chinese cosmology, the vagaries of the weather (*qixiang* 气象), the physical bearing of a person (*qise* 气色) or losing one's temper (*shengqi* 生气), among others.

In TCM theory, *qi* has a number of specific medical meanings depending on the context in which the term is used. In general, when we talk about *qi* in TCM, we have in mind a certain physiological function inside the body, or a substance that has a particular function. In other words, *qi* sometimes refers to a substance, and other times to a physiological function. TCM theory does not deal with the question of transferring *qi* from one person to another. Some practitioners of *qigong* healing and Chinese martial arts are believed to be able to transfer some kind of life force (also termed "*qi*") to other people for tonic and healing purposes. Conventional TCM theory is silent on this matter.

Whatever gets transferred in *qigong* healing may not necessarily be the same *qi* that TCM theory deals with.

A comprehensive discourse on the nature and functions of *qi* would take a whole scholarly volume by itself. For the purpose of this book, we look at three major categories of *qi* in TCM theory:

1. *Qi* as a substance that is vital to life. It can be transported through the meridians to the body's organs, some of which are able to store it like a chemical fuel.
2. *Qi* as energy. Lay expositions of Chinese medicine that translate *qi* as "vital energy" largely have this meaning in mind. This energy drives the function of our vital organs, propels blood and helps move and transform food in the body's digestive process. Acupuncture can be used to stimulate the flow of this vital energy.
3. *Qi* as a kind of physiological capability in the body. There are a multitude of such capabilities, such as the ability of the body to defend against harmful climatic influences like cold and wind, the ability to fight off invasions of external pathogens, the ability of the lung to breathe and project voice, and the ability of the body to contain or hold back excessive sweating, prolapse leading to hernias, and leakage of fluid from blood vessels.

According to Chinese medical theory, we are all born with a certain amount of *qi* from our parents, stored in the kidney at birth. Healthy parents and good care and nutrition for the mother during pregnancy ensure more abundant *qi* stored in the child's kidney at birth. After birth, the child acquires more *qi* from food, air and exercise, and this is stored in the various organs in the body.

Among the daily physiological functions of *qi* are the following:

- The propelling function that drives blood, enables fluid passage within the body, and is the moving force behind digestion.
- The warming function, as *qi* is a source of heat for the body, carrying nourishment with it for body tissues, which explains why an inadequate level of *qi* can lead to cold hands and feet.
- The protective function, with circulating *qi* at the surface level of the body acting like protective armour against the invasion of external pathogens such as wind and cold.
- The fixating or consolidating (固摄) function, where *qi* keeps fluids within blood vessels and tissues; it prevents excessive loss of fluids by sweating and loss of blood through oozing out of blood vessels.
- The transforming function, with *qi* converting food into a kind of essence (气化), transforming one kind of fluid into another, as well as helping with the excretion of waste substances.
- The transmitting function, where *qi* carries emotional signals from the mind to an associated organ, such as anger being transmitted to the liver. (This relationship between emotions and internal organs is very important in TCM theory and will be discussed further.)

The term "***zheng qi***" (正气) is associated with the vital functions of protecting the body against external pathogens that cause disease as well as the ability of the body to recover from illness; hence, it has commonality with the Western medical concept of the body's immune system, but with much wider application. It is variously translated as "genuine *qi*", "vital *qi*" and "**healthy *qi***". The *Neijing* aphorism "*zheng qi cun nei , xie bu ke* *gan*" (正气存内，邪不可干) means that if there is sufficient healthy *qi* in the body, it will not succumb to external pathogens.

Whilst "*zheng qi*" is a general term used to characterize a healthy body, there are various classifications of *qi* in the Chinese medical literature to describe more specific capabilities. Apart from *qi* associated with the proper functioning of each internal organ, there are four principal kinds of *qi* that are associated with the normal functioning of the body:

- **Primordial *qi* or *yuan qi* (元气):** This is inherited from parents and stored in the kidney; it is supplemented with air, nourishment and exercise and is an important reservoir of *qi* in the human body. In situations of extreme stress and damage to the body through illness, *yuan qi* is depleted; its restoration then becomes an important step to health recovery.
- **Pectoral *qi* or *zong qi* (宗气):** This is the *qi* stored in the thoracic area. It warms the vessels and nourishes the lung; an abundance of it gives a person a sonorous voice that is good for public speaking and singing.
- **Nutrient *qi* or *ying qi* (营气):** This circulates in the body and nourishes the internal organs.
- **Defensive *qi* or *wei qi* (卫气):** This *qi* moves in the outer layer of the body and defends it against external pathogens. When the body's defensive *qi* is weak, it is more vulnerable to harmful forces like cold, wind, dampness and heat. Defensive *qi* also helps regulate sweat to maintain body temperature.

2.3.1.2. *Blood*

Blood in TCM is similar to that in Western medicine but has a somewhat wider meaning. It is closely related to *qi*. In TCM, blood is produced by essence (*jing* 精) in the kidney and essence derived from food nutrients; *qi* participates in the transformation of essence into blood.

The functions of blood in TCM theory are to nourish and moisten the body. Since blood contains nutrient *qi*, it can nourish all the organs in the body. The fluid in blood moistens the vital organs as well as the orifices and joints. Blood also transports turbid *qi* to the lung where it is excreted by respiration.

Blood flow in the body is propelled by the *qi* of the heart. If the heart *qi* is inadequate, the blood will become too weak to circulate and this can have an impact on the working of the mind by causing conditions like insomnia. Other internal organs like the lung, spleen and liver are also involved in the circulation of blood. The lung is thought to be connected to all vessels of the body (hence the aphorism "the lung faces all vessels 肺朝百脉"); it accumulates *qi* and blood from the whole body to assist the heart to propel blood circulation. The spleen "commands" blood, directing it to circulate normally and preventing it from flowing out of the blood vessels. The liver stores blood and regulates the volume of blood, smoothing the activity of *qi* to promote blood circulation.

Factors that can affect blood circulation are the state of the vessels and changes in temperature. Phlegm, dampness, blood stasis, swellings and nodules can also obstruct blood circulation.

Blood and *qi* are so closely related that they are almost like two sides of the same coin. TCM theory puts it this way: "Blood is the mother of *qi* and *qi* is the marshall of blood" (血为气之母, 气为血之帅). Blood carries *qi* and is also essential to the production of *qi* by providing nutrients to the vital organs and the meridians. *Qi* is the driving force that enables blood circulation; as we noted earlier, *qi* also plays a role in the production of blood.

2.3.1.3. *Body fluids*

Body fluids (*jinye* 津液) help maintain life activities in the body. The main component of body fluids is water, which contains nutrient substances and is a component of blood in the blood vessels. Body fluids also flow outside the vessels in the vital organs and in the rest of the body. They can be excreted as tears, nasal discharges, tears and saliva. Among the functions of body fluids are moistening and nourishing, and the transportation of turbid *qi* for excretion.

2.3.2. Channels and collaterals

Channels (meridians) and collaterals (*jingluo* 经络) are the pathways along which travel *qi*, nutrients and messages linking the mind to the various organs. Channels are the main trunks while collaterals are the branches. Together they form an important network for the proper functioning of the body. Acupuncture needles are used at specific points (*xuewei* 穴位) in this network, promoting the flow of *qi* to relieve blockages to stimulate particular organs.

The principal components of the network are the twelve channels and eight extraordinary vessels (*qijing bamai* 奇经八脉). Each channel is associated with a particular organ, while the extraordinary vessels have no direct connection to the organs. Of the eight extraordinary vessels, the most commonly used ones for acupuncture are the governor vessel (*dumai* 督脉), the conception vessel (*renmai* 任脉) and the thoroughfare vessel (*chongmai* 冲脉).

The relevance of the channels and collateral network to cancer therapy lies in the association of these channels to particular organs, or to specific functions and parts of the body. For example, acupuncture needles applied to the spleen and stomach channels can have a tonifying effect on these organs. Cancer patients often suffer from deficiency of *qi* in the spleen and stomach, and acupuncture can be used together with herbal medications to strengthen these organs.

2.3.3. The organ systems

In accordance with the Chinese medical classification, the body's organs are divided into five solid storage organs known as *zang* 脏 and six hollow organs known as *fu* 腑. They are paired up as shown in Table 2.1.

The *zang* organs are regarded as solid as they have storage functions, including the storage of *qi* and essence. The *fu* organs are hollow in the sense that substances pass through them, as in the case of food passing through the stomach and the intestines. They are paired in the sense that they usually act in concert and support one another. For example, the spleen and stomach are both involved in digestion, and are often referred to together as *piwei* 脾胃; likewise, the kidney and bladder act together, one processing and the other holding urine before it is excreted. A sixth *fu* organ, not listed, is known as *sanjiao* 三焦 or the "triple

Table 2.1.   **Pairing of *Zang* and *Fu* Organs.**

Zang	Fu
Liver (*gan* 肝)	Gallbladder (*dan* 胆)
Heart (*xin* 心)	Small intestine (*xiaochang* 小肠)
Spleen (*pi* 脾)	Stomach (*wei* 胃)
Lung (*fei* 肺)	Large intestine (*dachang* 大肠)
Kidney (*shen* 肾)	Bladder (*pangguang* 膀胱)

energizer", which is essentially the trunk of the body from thorax to abdomen divided into three sections. It does not pair with any of the *zang* organs.

It is important to understand that organs in TCM are *not* the same as the organs with the same names in Western anatomy. *Each organ in TCM represents a set of functions.* In Western anatomy, an organ refers to a physical entity that can be identified at a fixed position in the body. A TCM organ, on the other hand, is physically less well defined. It is the traditional Chinese medical way of clustering a set of physiological functions so that all the main functions of the body can be captured by the five *zang* and six *fu* organs. Put in a different way, an organ in TCM is really a set of functions clustered in such a way to fit TCM models of health and physiology. This often causes considerable confusion to readers of Chinese medical literature who have not been exposed to the theory and models of TCM. We describe briefly the main functions of the five *zang* organs as employed in TCM theory.

The kidney (*shen*) has functions far beyond those of excretion. It is involved in growth, development, sex and reproduction, keeping the body warm, the production of bone marrow and brain matter, and the maintenance of the body's immune system. Hence, when a TCM physician speaks of a weak kidney, he is not necessarily referring to the person's problem with urination, but quite possibly to such unrelated problems as low libido or inability to withstand cold.

The spleen or *pi* in TCM represents, among other things, a set of digestive functions such that the whole digestive process is associated with the *piwei* (spleen and stomach). As the digestive function is at the base of serving nutrition to the other organs and all tissues of the body, the spleen is vital to the healthy functioning of the body and a precondition for restoring health to other organs that may have been injured or weakened by illness. It is therefore the main organ that replenishes primordial *qi* (*yuan qi*) in the kidney; hence, the spleen is sometimes known as the foundation of body health after birth (*hou tian zhi ben* 后天之本). Renowned physician Li Dongyuan of the Song dynasty paid great attention to the spleen in therapy and based much of his medical skills on the management of the spleen function, as described in his medical classic *Treatise on the Spleen and Stomach* that has been a reference manual for generations of Chinese physicians after him up to the present day. The spleen in TCM also "commands" blood (统血) in the sense of controlling blood circulation within the blood vessels and preventing it from flowing out of the vessels.

The principal activity of the liver in TCM is to "dredge and regulate" (疏泄), which is the idea of "dredging" the routes along which *qi* flows, and at the same time regulating the flow and activity of *qi*. It is a somewhat special concept peculiar to TCM, not found in Western medicine. In Chinese therapy involving improving this liver function, the term "*shugan*" (疏肝, literally meaning "dredging and regulating the liver") is frequently used. In this book, we choose "soothing the liver" as a more appropriate translation.

By regulating the activity of *qi*, the liver also regulates the activities of all other vital organs and tissues. Among the implications of this main function of the liver is that it promotes circulation of blood and metabolism in the body, and also assists the spleen and stomach in digestion. As is the case for the liver in Western medical anatomy, the liver in TCM also stores blood.

The heart in TCM has two main functions: to "govern" blood and to control the mind. The first function is similar to the heart function in Western medical physiology in the sense that it propels blood to circulate in the vessels; but it also has the implication that the heart is involved in the production of blood. The second function implies that the heart stores the "spirit", which has the function of cognition, consciousness and mental states. In this sense, the function of the heart in TCM includes some of the key functions of the brain in Western medical physiology.

The lung has the function of governing *qi* by controlling respiratory movement as well as controlling and regulating *qi* activities in the body, including the production of pectoral *qi* (*zong qi*) that we described earlier in the section on different kinds of *qi*. The lung also regulates water passages in the body for transmitting and discharging water, thereby propelling, adjusting and excreting water from the body. Another important aspect of the lung is that it assists the heart in blood circulation as in TCM theory blood from vessels converges in the lung and is redistributed to the rest of the body. This is the rationale behind the *Neijing*'s famous aphorism that "the lung is connected to all blood vessels" (肺朝百脉). One possible implication of this for the understanding of lung cancer is that a malignant tumour in the lung tends to spread to most parts of the body. In practice, we do observe that late-stage lung cancer is accompanied by spread to such diverse places as the bones, brain, liver and brain.

In this book, we use organ names in both the TCM and Western ways, and it should be clear from the context which of these is the subject under discussion. For example, when we speak of cancer of the lung or of the liver, we are referring to the physical lung and liver as in Western anatomy. However, when we are describing Chinese medications for deficiencies in the *qi* of the spleen, treating certain pathological conditions arising from cancer of the lung, it would be clear that we are referring to the TCM spleen and not the spleen of Western anatomy. The reader will notice in Chapters 3 and 4 that much of TCM therapy for cancer patients revolve around stomach-spleen organs and the kidney used in the TCM sense.

A comprehensive discussion of the functions within TCM theory of the five *zang* and six *fu* organs is outside the scope of this introduction to TCM diagnosis and treatment. For more on the TCM theory of organs or *zangxiang* theory (藏象学说), one of the textbooks in the References section of the book[12] can be consulted.

2.4. Models for Analysis and Diagnosis of Illness

TCM theory makes use of a number of models in a similar manner to the use of models in modern science to describe physical phenomena to make it easier for people to visualize and understand them. For example, physics theory pictures gases in an enclosed chamber as comprising molecules in rapid motion like billiard balls bouncing off the walls of the vessel. Economic science depicts an economy as comprising numerous individuals acting as if they were constantly maximizing an entity called "utility", a kind of usefulness and satisfaction that they seek primarily. Market demand and supply equations and the theory of the firm are built on this basic picture, taking into account constraints of time and physical resources.

In the case of TCM, the situation is somewhat fuzzier. This is because early medical thinkers also believed in cosmological theories of how the universe was formed and cosmic relations among stars in the heaven, and among elements on earth, and borrowed generously from these ancient models to try to understand the functioning of the human body. One result of this was that the body was viewed as a microcosm of the universe, that is, the rules that govern the external universe apply equally within the human

---

[12] Chai (2007); Wu (2002).

body. While we know now that many of these models on which
TCM was partly based are not appropriate for describing the
physical world, the fact remains that the TCM models derived
from them have gone through many changes over hundreds of
years so as to fit empirical observations from the medical records
and clinical work of generations of physicians. One can reasona-
bly take the view that it does not matter how the early versions of
these models were originally made up in ancient times. What matters is whether the empirically based models later used by Chinese
medicine provide good explanations of medical observations and
provide useful guides to choosing appropriate therapies for medical conditions.

In other words, the models used as a guide to diagnosis and
therapy by modern TCM physicians are heuristic models that have
been found from experience (mainly clinical work and recorded
case studies) to work well enough to be retained and employed by
the profession. We discuss here some of the models used regularly
in TCM diagnosis and therapy. Admittedly, the models used in
TCM have not been subjected to the same level of rigour in clinical
trials as is now customary in modern Western medicine.
Nevertheless, an increasing amount of scientific work is being
undertaken in universities and research institutions in China and
many other countries, including those in the West, to establish the
usefulness and validity of these models.

2.4.1. The *yin-yang* model

The *yin-yang* model describes many entities and states of the
world in terms of a duality, *yin* and *yang*. Thus, night is *yin*, day
is *yang*; female is *yin* and male is *yang*; soft, wetness, darkness and
obscurity are *yin* characteristics, whilst hardness, dryness, bright-
ness and transparency are *yang*. Looked at this way, the *yin-yang*
duality is simply a common-sense way of categorizing opposing

characteristics. Applied to medical concepts, we classify heat as associated with *yang* and cold with *yin*, *qi* with *yang* and blood with *yin*, and so on.

One of the fundamental principles of the *yin-yang* model is that in a healthy human body, *yin* and *yang* are in harmony and in balance: the body is neither hot nor cold, nor is it in a state of "excess" or "deficiency"; body fluids flow smoothly instead of being in a state of stagnation. Balance implies that pairs of opposite forces are in equilibrium, a little like homeostasis in Western medicine. *Yin* and *yang* are opposed but in a harmonious coalition with each other: *yin* representing darker, cooler and more flexible forces; *yang* representing brighter, warmer and more rigid forces. The body is neither hot nor cold; there is no excess or deficiency of energy; and all fluids flow smoothly without obstruction. Illness sets in when there is imbalance and therapy consists of restoring balance.

2.4.2. Causes of illness

TCM does not focus on germs like viruses and bacteria or cellular disorders as the causes of disease, and instead places more emphasis on fundamental factors in the external as well as the body's internal environment as the root causes. This does not mean that TCM does not acknowledge the role of germs and cellular disorders in bringing about disease or affecting its progression, but rather it views the external and internal environmental factors (pathogens) as playing a more basic role.

Among these pathogenic factors, six exogenous (climatic) factors and seven internal emotional factors are commonly identified. Modern TCM texts also factor in toxic chemicals, microbiological agents (viruses, bacteria, fungi, etc) and parasites. Although recognizing the role of these microbiological and other agents, TCM theory defers to Western medicine to deal with these matters and emphasizes the bigger holistic picture of how climatic and emotional factors and dietary and living habits provide the preconditions for the successful invasion of these agents into the body and their taking hold to bring about disease.

The **six exogenous factors** (六淫) are as follows:

1. wind (风);
2. cold (寒);
3. summer heat (暑);
4. dampness (湿);
5. dryness (燥);
6. fire (火).

When these climatic factors invade the body and are not expelled, they can become internal pathogenic factors as well with characteristics similar to their external counterparts. Wind is blamed for the largest variety of illnesses, hence the saying that "a hundred illnesses arise from wind" (风为百病之始). Wind is characterized by movement, hence when it is in the body the problem that it causes tends to move around. Thus, pain from rheumatism is thought to be due to movement of wind within the body. Wind can also be internally generated, for example by an overexuberant liver that causes wind to travel to the head, causing dizziness, hypertension and even a cerebral stroke.

Cold and heat in the weather have parallels internally in pathological conditions of heat and cold. Summer heat is associated with extreme heat (fire) and often with dampness as well.

Dampness is high humidity when it is external and is associated with symptoms of stickiness (clinging on and being difficult to eliminate) when it is internal, slowing a person down and causing stagnation in digestion when it is present in the spleen.

Dryness, on the other hand, is present typically in autumn and winter months in temperate countries and air-conditioned rooms in the tropics.

Besides these pathogens that are directly or indirectly related to climate, there are other internal pathogens, the main ones being phlegm (*tan* 痰) and toxins (*du* 毒). Phlegm in TCM refers not just to the sticky viscous substance that lines one's throat and bronchioles, causing irritation and coughing that tries to expel it, but also to the nasty clear fluids that inhabit the digestive system and other vital organs, causing ailments such as indigestion, lassitude, insomnia, irascible moods, headaches and strokes, earning it the aphorisms "百病多由痰作祟" (a hundred ailments are induced by phlegm) and "怪病多痰" (strange diseases are caused mainly by phlegm). Interestingly, phlegm also has mischievous roles to play in ancient Greco-Roman medicine: Legendary Roman physician Galen listed phlegm as one of the four humours alongside blood, choler and black bile, attributing one's temperament mainly to these humours, but did not give phlegm the wide and powerful influence it finds in TCM. Toxins are commonly found in TCM literature, with many herbs able to resolve toxins (*jie du* 解毒). In Chapter 4 of this book, you will come across many examples of accumulation of toxins associated with cancerous tumours, hence the elimination of toxins is an important part of cancer treatment in TCM.

The **seven emotions** (七情) in TCM are pleasure, anger, anxiety, grief, fear, shock and melancholy. The first five are more commonly encountered and each is associated with a specific *zang* organ (Table 2.2).

Pleasure refers to excessive indulgence in pleasurable activities, including excessive sex. Anger damages the liver, which explains why a sudden fit of anger can cause wind or fire to rise

Table 2.2.   The Seven Emotions and the Associated Organs.

Emotion	Organ Damaged by Emotion
Pleasure 喜	Heart
Anger 怒	Liver
Anxiety 思	Spleen
Grief 悲	Lung
Fear 恐	Kidney
Shock 惊	Heart
Melancholy 忧	Lung, liver

from the liver to the head and cause headaches, dizziness, red eyes or elevated blood pressure. Anxiety (sometimes also just termed "thinking" or "contemplation"), on the other hand, acts slowly on the spleen, gnawing away at one's health at the basic level of digestion and nutrition. It is the most insidious and damaging form of emotion, wearing down the body and eventually leading to more serious illnesses as the other organs are affected by the poor functioning of the spleen. Irritable bowel syndrome, accompanied by such symptoms as a bloated abdomen, loose stools, indigestion and loss of appetite, is regarded to be caused mainly by disorder of the spleen function. In social environments where there is a high and sustained level of stress in everyday living, one tends to see more illnesses related to the spleen with the underlying cause of anxiety. Grief damages the lung, and TCM postulates that this is the reason we sigh a lot when stricken with grief. Fear affects the kidney, and is thought to be the reason that extreme fear can cause incontinence and could also affect reproductive fertility.

2.4.3. Differentiating syndromes and applying therapy

Differentiating syndromes and applying treatment accordingly (*bianzheng lunzhi* 辨证论治) is a distinguishing feature of TCM theory and is a core part of the Chinese holistic approach to health and healing.

A syndrome or *zheng* (证) in TCM refers to a pattern of symptoms associated with a pathological process; it has a slightly similar meaning but really quite different conceptual base from that of the same term used in Western medicine. The latter uses the term to refer to "a combination of signs and/or symptoms that forms a distinct clinical picture indicative of a particular disorder".[13] Common Western medical syndromes include irritable bowel syndrome, Down's syndrome and acquired immunodeficiency syndrome (AIDS).

The syndrome in TCM is a concept closely bound with the Chinese medical models of *yin-yang*, organ systems and internal pathogens. The syndrome is also different from disease (*bing* 病), which comprises a group of symptoms with a coherent and recurring aetiology such as to be found in diseases like tuberculosis, gastric ulcers or diabetes. A syndrome is a picture or manifestation of a pathological condition of the body. Simple syndromes would be such conditions as deficiency (**asthenic**) syndrome, excess (**sthenic**) syndrome, heat, cold, dampness, wind, phlegm, blood stasis and *qi* and/or blood stagnation. Usually a deficiency or excess would be of *yin*, *yang*, *qi* or blood of *qi*. Typically we would speak of an excess of heat, or a deficiency of *yin* or *yang*.

More complex syndromes would involve particular organs or a combination of a number of syndromes. For example, a deficiency

---

[13] *Oxford Concise Medical Dictionary* (2007).

in the *qi* of the spleen would be referred to as "deficiency of spleen *qi*". If the *yang* of the liver is in excess and there is at the same time *qi* stagnation in the liver, the complex syndrome would be called "excess of liver *yang* with *qi* stagnation".

Many diseases can exhibit the same syndrome at a particular phase of the development of the disease. Cancer is a disease, but at various stages of the development of the disease, one can observe *qi* deficiency of the spleen, heat in the liver or deficiency in kidney *yin*. TCM therapy is aimed at reducing or eliminating these syndromes as an integral part of alleviating the symptoms of the disease and eliminating the disease. It should now be quite clear why the same syndrome can be found in many diseases. For example, *qi* weakness is seen in coronary heart disease as well as stomach ulcers. A disease is usually in a dynamic state. In the course of its progression (called "pathogenesis") it can exhibit different syndromes. For example, tuberculosis is a disease with symptoms of coughing up blood, daily fever, lassitude and loss of weight. A person with the disease would exhibit different TCM syndromes at different stages of its progression such as *qi* stagnation in the stomach/spleen, followed by deficiency of kidney *yang*, and would therefore require a different treatment regimen at each stage.

2.4.4. Diagnostic model of the four examinations

TCM diagnosis is largely about determining the syndromes present in the body at a given time. This is achieved by the classical method of the four examinations (*si zhen* 四诊 or *wang wen wen qie* 望闻问切) comprising the following:

1. visual observation (望);
2. listening and olfaction (闻);

3. inquiry (问);
4. pulse-taking and palpation (切).

The basic principle of the four examinations is to make inferences about the body's internal condition based on symptoms observable by the physician. In ancient times, the physician did not have diagnostic tools like X-rays, laboratory blood tests, ultrasound and MRI that are now the common fare of Western physicians. The modern TCM physician continues in the tradition of the ancients by relying on the four examinations to detect external symptoms that allow him to draw conclusions about the patient's *syndromes*. This is akin to a mapping process, where each observation determines the locus of one aspect of the patient's condition. From the overall map that is presented after completing the four examinations, there is usually sufficient information for the experienced physician to draw a conclusion about the patient's internal condition. We briefly describe here some of the main features in the application of the four examinations.

2.4.4.1. *Visual observation*

The patient's face is observed in detail for such manifestations as the colour of the skin, the presence or absence of a healthy glow, the spirit in his eyes (whether full of life, dispirited, filled with anger or sadness, etc) and the presence of unusual growths or pigmentation of the skin. The patient's manner of walking is also observed as he walks into the physician's clinic, and anything unusual in his posture and gait is noted. His whole body is also examined if the physician feels that is necessary.

The examination of the tongue is an extremely important part of the visual observation. Several aspects of the tongue are noted: its size (whether thin and withered, or swollen with tooth indentations, or normal), its colour and, very significantly, the texture and the colour of the fur on the tongue. A slightly red tongue is normal but a deeper red could indicate internal heat, whilst a dark tongue with a purplish hue is often associated with poor blood circulation and blood stasis.

A person of normal health would have thin whitish fur on the tongue. Thick greasy fur indicates the presence of dampness, while unusually thin fur, or no fur at all, can imply the presence of *yin* deficiency resulting in asthenic internal heat. Thick yellow-ish fur is usually associated with internal heat resulting from an excess syndrome.

2.4.4.2. *Listening and olfaction*

The physician listens to the patient's voice to determine if it is weak or strong, smooth or hoarse, clear or slurred. His manner of breathing, whether slow or hurried, smooth or laboured, shallow or deep, and the presence of cough are all noted. Olfaction, or detecting unusual odours from the body, is also part of the examination process.

2.4.4.3. *Inquiry*

For the first visit to a physician, the patient should be asked a long list of questions concerning his past medical history, bowel movements, urination, appetite, sleep, adaptability to hot and cold environments, aversion to wind, sexual activities, eyesight and moods. This could take 15 to 30 minutes depending on the complexity of the patient's condition. Of course, he is also asked to describe how he feels, and the main medical complaint that led him to consult the physician.

An experienced physician can ask searching and penetrating questions that allow him to accurately narrow down the range of conditions with which the patient might be afflicted. In a sense, the inquiry part of the four examinations is the most challenging but also the most rewarding one as a tremendous amount of information can be extracted from this process. Modern Western doctors who rely heavily on laboratory diagnostic tests and spend less time understanding how the patient feels could be missing crucial information that can help the doctor determine the patient's condition.

2.4.4.4. *Pulse-taking and palpation*

There is a popular belief about Chinese physicians that a good one can know everything about a patient by taking his pulse. There are even stories of physicians who took pulses by tying a string to the patient's wrist and detecting his pulse through the string without touching the patient, then going on to make an accurate diagnosis of the patient's condition. Legend has it that the queen and concubines of a Chinese emperor cannot be physically touched by the royal physician who therefore has to rely on this unusually discreet method of pulse-taking.

The practical truth is that the pulse is but only one indicator of the patient's condition. Although an important indicator, it need not be the most crucial one; neither is it normally sufficient to allow the physician to determine accurately the syndromes present in the patient.

Nevertheless it cannot be denied that pulse-taking is a crucial part of the examination process for a patient. TCM differentiates between dozens of different pulses, determined by placing three fingers on the patient's wrist (left and right in turn). Some of the common types of pulses encountered in

Table 2.3.   Types of Pulses and Their Indications.

Type of Pulse	Indication
Floating pulse (浮脉)	External syndrome, near skin level
Sunken pulse (沉脉)	Internal syndrome, deeper in the body
Moderately slow pulse (缓脉)	Dampness and weakness in spleen/stomach
Fast pulse (数脉)	Heat syndrome
Weak pulse (虚脉)	Asthenic syndrome, usually in *qi* and blood
Feeble pulse (弱脉)	Decline in *qi* and blood
Powerful pulse (实脉)	Sthenic syndrome
Slippery pulse (滑脉)	Retention of phlegm and fluid; sthenic heat
Thready pulse (细脉)	Asthenia of *qi* and blood
Taut pulse (弦脉)	Phlegm; liver and gallbladder disorders
Tense pulse (紧脉)	Cold syndrome; food retention

clinical practice are listed in Table 2.3 together with their usual indications.

2.4.5. Principles of health and therapy in TCM

The concept of health in TCM derives from the *Neijing* notion that human bodies in harmonious balance — within the body as well as with their natural environments — do not fall ill. This is to a large extent consistent with the idea of evolutionary medicine that the human body is adapted to survive in its natural environment if it is protected against external pathogens by prudent living and maintains health internally by having proper control over diet, emotions, and adequate exercise. However, it has been pointed out by evolutionary biologists that the body is not perfect, and that evolution leaves some defects that sometimes result in disease, and that environmental changes can also trigger new disorders.[14]

When the body falls ill, TCM views it as the presence of one or more syndromes. Hence, the main principle of therapy is to resolve or eliminate the syndromes so that the body returns as close as possible to its natural healthy state of being in internal balance and in harmony with its environment. It is in this sense that TCM is said to be holistic: its diagnostic and therapeutic methods attempt to look at the body as a whole in terms of internal and external harmony. The principle of therapy is therefore deceptively simple: restore the body as close as possible to its normal state by alleviating or eliminating as many syndromes as possible present. Unlike Western medicine, TCM does not specifically try to attack germs present or kill off diseased cells (such as cancer cells). Instead, it tries to restore balance, and when that is achieved the germs and diseased cells are either destroyed or kept under control so that the body functions normally. The combination of TCM and Western medical therapies can potentially achieve the best results: it addresses the imbalances at the holistic level and uses the tremendous curative arsenal of Western medicine to attack disease-causing agents and diseased cells. Many examples of this combined approach to cancer therapy will be covered in Chapters 3 and 4.

The principle of TCM therapy targeted at syndromes is relatively straightforward: combat the syndrome with the opposite force or countervailing measure. When there is heat, we cool the body or dissipate the heat; when there is cold, we warm it; when there is stagnation of *qi* or blood, we promote flow; when there is deficiency or weakness in the *qi* of a particular organ, we

---

[14] See, for example, Neese and Williams (1996).

strengthen or tonify the *qi* of that organ; when there is phlegm, we use phlegm-clearing drugs to resolve it; when there is dampness, we dry the body by expelling dampness; when there is wind, we quell or calm the wind with wind-resolving medications. Simple as these measures may sound, it takes an experienced and skilful physician to diagnose the symptoms and decide which ones to treat with higher priority and to select the combination of herbs, acupuncture and other therapy modalities that would best achieve these results, taking into account the individual constitution and condition of the patient at any particular time. As the case studies in Chapter 5 will show, cancer patients usually have a variety of syndromes simultaneously present and are also weakened by surgery, chemotherapy or radiotherapy, so they are not always able to tolerate or benefit from common herbs used to treat particular syndromes. The judgement and experience of the attending physician is then of particular importance.

There are four principal modes of therapy in Chinese medicine: herbs, acupuncture, *tuina* (medical massage) and *qigong*. These are used either singly or in combination, depending on the condition of the patient and the resources available.

Herbs and acupuncture are the most common modes, often used together, one reinforcing the other or covering an aspect of therapy for which it is more appropriate. For example, a person with back pain caused by strain or trauma to the back muscle or the spinal vertebra could be administered acupuncture to improve *qi* and blood circulation in the affected areas; this can be supplemented by herbs that promote circulation and remove blood stasis. In this case, herbs and acupuncture complement and reinforce each other. On the other hand, a person suffering from a respiratory infection and has a running nose and cough would benefit from acupuncture in the nasal, chest and certain acupuncture points on his arms to relieve nasal congestion. But acupuncture is not as effective for the elimination of heat and clearing of phlegm in his chest. This is better achieved with cooling herbs such as *Ge Gen* (葛根) and *Ju Hua* (chrysanthemum) and phlegm-resolving herbs such as *Ban Xia* (半夏) and *Chen Pi* (陈皮).

Tuina is closely related to acupuncture as it works on the same points and meridians as acupuncture, except that instead of needles, the hands and fingers of the therapist are employed. *Tuina* has the advantage of being non-invasive and more comfortable for some people than acupuncture needles. It can also be more effective than acupuncture for certain muscular and joint conditions.

Qigong involves, among other things, the promotion of *qi* generation and *qi* flow in the body. There are two main types: dynamic (moving) *qigong* (动功) and quiescent *qigong* (静功). The former is practised by movement of the body and limbs, combined with suitable breathing; the latter is centred on focusing the mind through meditation and breathing techniques.

All modes of therapy are potentially useful for cancer patients, although there is a predominance of herbal medicine. The use of acupuncture and *qigong* may be appropriate in the recovery phase for cancer cases (see, for example, Case 2 on lung cancer in Chapter 5).

2.5. TCM as Science

Is TCM a science? A person trained in modern physical and biological sciences could be forgiven for dismissing any claim that TCM makes to being a science. To start with, many of the concepts and entities that form the basis of TCM theory are not measurable or even detectable by scientific instruments. For example, *qi* has never been captured in a bottle for chemical analysis, nor has the phlegm that causes a multitude of disorders in the body been isolated and its physical properties observed and recorded. With regard to TCM therapeutic methods, while there are many recorded case studies of physicians who healed patients using the principle of differentiating syndromes, very little has been done by way of large-scale clinical trials that are expected in evidence-based Western medicine.

Nevertheless there is a sense in which TCM is similar to the physical and biological sciences: it is based on empirical observations and inferences drawn from these observations. TCM theory uses complex concepts like *qi* and phlegm and a simplified picture of the human body comprising a few organs and a network of meridians. It can be interpreted as having invented these concepts and entities in order to explain the behaviour of the body in a way that makes them useful for diagnosis and healing. It sets out a set of principles of diagnosis and therapy by differentiating syndromes based on these pictures of the human body and models for the behaviour of these fluids, organs and meridians. These principles are tested each time a physician applies them to diagnose and treat a patient. Over thousands of years, these principles have been modified and refined to fit clinical experience.[15]

Hence, we can regard TCM entities and models as useful analogies and convenient constructs, heuristic in nature, based on the best fit they can make to empirical experience of treating illnesses. They are not to be understood literally and are more correctly regarded as useful tools for the purpose of using herbs, acupuncture and other therapies to help people overcome their illnesses and achieve a state of health. TCM is a science in this somewhat narrow and limited sense. In the tradition of Chinese

---

[15] See Hong (2009) for a comparison of the paradigms of Chinese and Western medicines.

pragmatism, what the underlying correct picture of the human body is not as important as whether or not this body of theory works as a system of medicine. In the words of the greatest pragmatist of modern China, Deng Xiaoping, what matters is not whether a cat is black or white, but whether it can catch mice. The history of Chinese medicine and the accumulated wisdom of physicians over thousands of years suggest that Chinese medicine is by no means perfect and cannot always be relied on to work, but that it has worked better in some areas than in others. Where it has worked, it has been able to play a significant and useful role in health care up to the present day. The effectiveness of TCM as complementary and alternative therapy to Western medicine in cancer management is one instance of the continuing usefulness of this method of healing.

CHAPTER 3

HERBS AND PRESCRIPTIONS FOR THERAPY

Of the four principal modes of therapy in Chinese medicine, namely herbs, acupuncture, *tuina* and *qigong*, the first is by far the most common modality used as herbs are easily accessible and can be boiled in the convenience of the home and readily consumed at appropriate times. In this chapter we discuss the use of Chinese herbs in general for health promotion and medical therapy. This serves as background information and knowledge for understanding the remainder of the book in which frequent reference will be made to prescriptions using Chinese herbs.

3.1. Chinese *Materia Medica*

In this book, we have used the common term "Chinese herbs" to refer to the whole range of natural materials that are used in Chinese medications. The correct term for these materials is "*materia medica*" as Chinese medical materials are derived not just from plants, but also animal parts and minerals. For convenience we henceforth simply use the term "herbs" to refer to *materia medica*.

Medicinal herbs have been used in Chinese medical practice for health promotion and treatment of illnesses for thousands of years. The properties and nature of these herbs and their therapeutic effects have been carefully studied and documented by over a hundred generations of herbalists and physicians. The earliest extant manual on herbs was written by the legendary Shennong of the Western Han dynasty (201 BC to 24 AD) in the classic *Shennong Herbal Manual* (神农本草经). This contained detailed descriptions of 365 herbs which he had come across in his travels across fields and mountains all over the country. Shennong personally tested these herbs on himself for toxicity and side effects at considerable risk to his life and health. During the Ming dynasty in 1578, the most comprehensive record of Chinese herbs to date was compiled, which has since served as a reference text for Chinese physicians and pharmacists. The *Compendium of Materia Medica* or *Bencao gangmu* (本草纲目) covered 1892 herbs (inclusive of those of animal and mineral origins). The encyclopaedic nature of these scholarly works testifies to the empirical scientific tradition in Chinese medicine which relies on clinical evidence provided by detailed observation, record and analysis.

In modern times, most of these herbs have been analysed in the laboratory and in clinical trials for therapeutic properties, toxicity and side effects and the accumulation of these studies and the experience of earlier generations of physicians have been carefully documented in modern texts on Chinese medicinal herbs. Much work remains to be done because the variety of herbs is very large and their complexity of a much higher order of magnitude as each herb contains dozens and sometimes over a hundred different ingredients and kinds of molecules in contrast to Western drugs that mainly comprise a single molecule for each drug. Some aspects of using Chinese herbs are worthy of note and we briefly describe them here.

3.2. Preparation and Consumption of Herbs for Medicinal Use

Boiling is the most common way of extracting medical ingredients from herbs, and the resultant liquid medicine is known as a decoction (tang 汤). The standard procedure for decoction is to boil the herbs for about 45 minutes, initially with high heat followed by moderate heat, using enough water to get one bowl. After that the same herbs should be boiled for 30 to 45 minutes for a second extraction, yielding a second (more diluted) bowl. Finally, the two bowls are mixed and separated again into two bowls of even concentration, for use within a single day. In some cases, the prescription may require using the decoction three times a day, in which case more water should be used to yield three bowls.

While this is the standard procedure, one has to take into account certain herbs that contain volatile ingredients, such as *Bo He* (薄荷) and *Xiang Fu* (香附), which should be added and boiled for only 10 minutes or less at the end of the second boil.

Besides decoctions, herbs can also be prepared to yield other forms for storage and consumption. Among these the powder (*san* 散) form is one of the most common, followed by pills and boluses. Medicinal ingredients in liquid form can also be extracted using alcohol in the form of Chinese white wine; these are particularly useful for tonic preparations.

The correct time to take herbal medications depends on the kind of medication, in particular whether or not they contain ingredients to which the stomach and the rest of the digestive system may be sensitive, such as herbs that are acidic in nature or are overly cool or warm in nature. Tonics are best ingested on an empty stomach before meals to ensure that the precious ingredients are better absorbed. Medicines that potentially irritate the digestive system are best taken after meals, whilst preparations for calming and tranquilizing effects are best taken at night before retiring to bed. Purgatives like *Da Huang* (大黄) should be avoided straight after or just before meals as the purging effect may interfere with the digestion of food and limit its absorption.

3.2.1. Processing of herbs

It should be noted that the processing of herbs can change the nature and properties of the herbs, so the use of some herbs should take into account the processing they have undergone before they are sold to the consumer. This helps to reduce toxicity and, sometimes changes its nature. Just as tea in mostly unprocessed form (like some green teas) can change its properties after processing by drying and warming, turning into a warmer and darker tea (like oolong or pu'er), so processing of herbs can also change their medicinal effects. For example, *Sheng Di Huang* (生地黄 raw rehmannia) is cold and bitter-sweet in nature and is used for clearing heat and cooling the blood, whereas the processed form *Shu Di Huang* (熟地黄) is warm and sweet and useful for enriching blood and nourishing *yin*.

3.3. Contraindications and Toxicities

Contraindications are conditions under which certain herbs may not be used or used only with caution and under proper medical instruction; this should be carefully observed when using herbs. Contraindications are well documented for all herbs in the Chinese pharmacopoeia. Many of these contraindications pertain to patients with weak or cold stomach/spleen symptoms, or have liver heat and wind disorders associated with high blood pressure, and to women who are pregnant or undergoing menses. For example, *She Xiang* (麝香) is known to be able to induce spontaneous abortion; *Chuan Wu* (川乌), *Chuan Xiong* (川芎) and *Hong Hua* (红花), all of which can remove blood stasis and improve blood circulation, should be used with caution by women who are pregnant or undergoing menses. American ginseng, (*Xi Yang Shen* 西洋参) is cool and can hurt the stomach and spleen of a patient with a weak or overly cool stomach.

Toxicity is a principal concern to users of Chinese herbs, particularly those in the West who have heard or read stories of the dangerous toxic effects of certain Chinese medicines. The true situation is that the toxicity of Chinese herbs and their side effects are well documented and the herbs can be safely used under competent medical guidance. In this regard, it is important to distinguish between two sources of toxicity:

1. Toxicity caused by impurities in the herbs. As herbs are mostly derived from the root, stem, bark, flower, seed and fruit of plants growing in the wild or under cultivation, impurities can enter through pollution in the atmosphere and soil. It would be fair to say that most Chinese herbs contain small albeit acceptable quantities of such impurities. The same applies to vegetables and fruits used in daily living throughout the world: much would depend on proper supervision of agriculture, the use of chemical fertilizers and the atmospheric and soil pollution in the regions where these foods are cultivated. Health and agricultural authorities usually require stringent checks to be made on the foods that are grown or imported for consumption. Unfortunately, the same level of rigour in supervising Chinese herbs has not been put in place in most countries.

Hence, it is important to obtain these herbs from reliable and reputable sources.

2. Natural toxicities of the herbs. As with Western drugs which have side effects, there are natural side effects or toxicities associated with some Chinese herbs. Most of these toxicities are not significantly harmful when the herbs are consumed in prescribed quantities; however, they are best used under the supervision of a physician who understands how they should be used and is able to provide guidance on the effects of these toxicities in the light of the condition of the patient. But it is generally true that because these herbs have been in use for hundreds, even thousands of years, their toxicities are well understood and documented in the Chinese pharmacopoeia, and there is very little risk associated with ingesting them under proper medical supervision.

The mutual **compatibility of herbs** should also be noted. Certain herbs can react with other drugs to cause undesired effects. Chinese medicine has identified these and listed them as the "18 incompatibilities" (*shibafan* 十八反). For example, *Ban Xia* is incompatible with *Wu Tou*, ginseng with *Li Lu*.

The interaction of Chinese herbs with Western drugs is not a well-researched area, and is a matter of concern to patients who are on Western medication and also wish to use some Chinese herbs. It is generally true that there are not many cases in which the interaction of common Chinese herbs with Western drugs becomes a significant problem but, as a precaution, patients are usually advised not to take them together or, if they should be taken together, that there be a two- to three-hour interval between taking Western and Chinese medicines. This unfortunately is not foolproof, as some Western drugs are active for much longer than three hours, particularly those that are controlled-release or sustained-release in design. As such, it is safer to consult competent physicians if the two kinds of medicine are taken together. One of the common areas of interaction is the use of blood thinners like aspirin and warfarin; it is generally inadvisable to take herbs in Chinese medicine that are classified as promoting blood circulation and removing blood stasis (*huoxue huayu* 活血化瘀), as the latter tend also to have a blood-thinning effect, thereby magnifying the blood-thinning effect of the Western drugs beyond a safe level.

In the case of cancer treatment with a combination of chemotherapy and Chinese herbs, Professor Yu's experience is that the herbs used for cancer management rarely ever interfere with chemotherapy. However, a word of caution may be in order as many new chemotherapy drugs are being introduced in the market at a rapid pace and there is no assurance that no incompatibility might occur in particular cases. As such, it would be prudent for the patient to keep the Western doctor informed of the Chinese herbs he is taking and follow advice from the doctor, or use them only when he is not undergoing chemotherapy.

3.4. Classification of Herbs

Herbs can be classified according to their natural characteristics, or according to their therapeutic effects.

3.4.1. Classification of herbs by natural characteristics

The **natural characteristics** of herbs include their properties, flavours and meridian tropism (归经), which is an indication of the meridians along which their therapeutic effects prefer to travel.

The **property** of a herb refers to its warming or cooling effect on the body. More specifically, herbs are classified as follows: hot, warm, neutral, cool and cold. As indicated in the last chapter, these warm and cool properties do not refer to their temperature but the effect on pathogenic heat and cold. Thus, peppermint and chrysanthemum are cool, whilst cinnamon and ginseng are warm. Herbs that are hot have stronger effects than warm herbs and can have more serious side effects like internal heat if taken in excess. Examples are *Fu Zi* and dried ginger. Conversely, herbs that are cold like gypsum and *Mu Dan Pi* (made from the root of the peony plant) are used to remove internal heat, but can have the side effects of harming the stomach and spleen if inappropriately used.

The **flavour** of a herb is akin to its taste, except that in Chinese medicine certain actions are associated with the flavour classification, hence there is not always an exact correspondence between flavour and taste. The five flavours are pungent (辛), sweet (甘), sour (酸), bitter (苦) and salty (咸), and their common actions are shown in Table 3.1.

Table 3.1.   The Five Flavours and Their Common Actions.

Flavour	Action	Example
Pungent	Dispersing and promoting circulation of *qi* and blood	*Bo He* (Herba Menthae)
Sweet	Nourishing, harmonizing and moistening	*Ginseng*
Sour	Absorbing, consolidating and astringent action	*Wu Mei* (dried plum)
Bitter	Drying or resolving dampness, purging	*Da Huang*
Salty	Softening hard nodes or masses and promoting defecation	*Mang Xiao*

Each herb is thought to have one or more preferential routes along the meridians for their actions to affect specific organs. Chrysanthemum and wolfberry seeds both prefer the liver meridian, and are often used in therapies involving the liver; they also have a preference for the lung meridian and are used in some cough medications.

3.4.2. Classification of herbs by therapeutic effects

Herbs are also classified according to their principal therapeutic effects. Some of the main classifications are as follows:

1. Diaphoretics (解表药): removing either warm or cold pathogens at the surface level.
2. Heat-clearing herbs (清热药): clearing internal heat.
3. Purgatives (泻下药): lubricating the last section of the intestine or inducing diarrhoea to move bowels and relieve constipation.
4. Dampness-removing herbs (祛湿药): eliminating dampness within the body and promoting diuresis.
5. Interior-warming herbs (温里药): warming the interior of the body and dispelling cold.
6. *Qi*-regulating herbs (理气药): promoting the movement of *qi*.
7. Herbs relieving food retention (消食药): helping with digestion and relieving food retention.
8. Haemostatic herbs (止血药): assisting in stopping bleeding internally and externally, by cooling the blood, warming the channels or astringent action.
9. Herbs invigorating the blood and removing stasis (活血化瘀药): promoting better blood flow and removing stasis.

10. Phlegm-resolving herbs (化痰药): removing phlegm in the body.
11. Tranquilizers (安神药): calming the mind.
12. Calming liver and wind (平肝熄风药): calming the liver and suppressing hyperactive *yang*, or calming liver wind.
13. Tonics (补益药): tonics for *qi*, blood, *yin* and *yang*.
14. Astringents (收敛固涩药): arresting discharge of excessive perspiration, diarrhoea, excessive urination, etc.

Although a herb may be classified according to its main action, most herbs have several other actions. This is because a herb contains a large variety of components and its action cannot be captured by just one classification. For example, wolfberry seeds or *Gou Qi Zi* (枸杞子) has the main therapeutic effect of tonifying the *yin* of the liver and kidney; it also improves the eyesight and also nourishes the lung.

A list of herbs used in the treatment of various conditions associated with cancer is provided in Appendix 1.

3.5. Chinese Medical Prescriptions

"*Fangji*" (方剂) is the TCM term for a medical prescription. The character "*fang*" (方) means "method"; in ordinary language, "*youfang*" (有方) means "having the right method, or the correct approach, to a problem". "*Ji*" means "medicine"; hence "*fangji*" denotes medicine formulated by a good method, i.e. a good prescription.

Chinese physicians have found over the years that herbs can be combined in a certain way to achieve the best desired result; much like a cocktail has a combination of ingredients to yield the best taste, or a food recipe to give us an appetizing and nutritious dish. Unlike Western medicine, Chinese prescriptions are customized for the individual, taking into account the type and severity of his syndromes as well as his constitution and state of health. However, Chinese medicine has developed over thousands of years also a number of standard prescriptions that can be used for patients falling within a category of syndromes. In practice, these standard or classical prescriptions can and often are modified by the physician to suit the individual.

These standard prescriptions are classified by therapeutic effect, similar to the way herbs are classified. Because the prescriptions contain several herbs, each playing a different role, a better result is usually obtained than by using just one herb. This is in contrast to Western drugs, each of which generally uses one molecule to act as the active ingredient, with other ingredients only providing a base for the delivery of that active ingredient. The general principle for combining herbs in Chinese medicine is based on one of four possible roles that each herb can play, namely the monarch, ministerial, adjuvant and guiding roles, also known as *jun* (君), *chen* (臣), *zuo* (佐) and *shi* (使) respectively.

1. The monarch or *jun* herb plays the core therapeutic role.
2. The ministerial or *chen* herb enhances the former's effect.
3. The adjuvant or *zuo* herb plays a complementary role, supporting the monarch herb by working on a related concomitant condition, or reducing toxicities and side effects, if any, of the monarch and ministerial herbs.
4. The guiding or *shi* herb helps direct the other herbs to the particular organs and harmonizes their joint action.

For example, the classical prescription called the Decoction of the Four Noble Herbs (*Si Jun Zi Tang* 四君子汤) contains ginseng (monarch herb), *Bai Zhu* 白术 (ministerial herb),

Fu Ling 茯苓 (adjuvant herb) and *Zhi Gan Cao* 炙甘草 (guiding herb). A common tonic for the spleen and stomach, this prescription replenishes *qi* and strengthens the spleen. It takes into account that spleen problems usually are accompanied by dampness. In this prescription, ginseng is a strong *qi* tonic, *Bai Zhu* is also a *qi* tonic that enhances ginseng's *qi*-replenishing action, whilst *Fu Ling* both adds to the *qi* tonic effect and removes dampness. *Zhi Gan Cao* harmonizes the combination; it is also in itself a mild *qi* and spleen tonic.

Not every prescription has herbs playing all four roles in combination. Many prescriptions have two or more herbs playing the same role. For example, the classic prescription Pill of Six Ingredients with Rehmannia (*Liu Wei Di Huang Wan* 六味地黄丸), a popular *yin* tonic for nourishing the kidney, comprises one monarch herb (rehmannia or *Shu Di Huang*), two ministerial herbs (*Shan Zhu Yu* and *Shan Yao*) and three adjuvant herbs (*Ze Xie, Mu Dan Pi* and *Fu Ling*). The monarch herb is a strong kidney tonic, whilst the two ministerial herbs also nourish the kidney, with *Shan Yao* also strengthening the spleen to complement the kidney function. The three adjuvant herbs play varying roles of reducing dampness, clearing heat arising from *yin* deficiency of the kidney and improving the transportation and transformation function of the spleen. In combination, they tonify the kidney and spleen as well as dissipate internal heat in a balanced and gentle manner, making it one of the most successful prescriptions in the history of Chinese medicine, used equally by physicians treating illnesses as well as the common man as a dietary supplement to combat the weakening of the kidney function that come with ageing and with daily stresses.

To customize a prescription, physicians often use one of the standard formulations and modify it to suit the individual's particular condition. For example, *Liu Wei Di Huang Wan* can be modified for someone with kidney *yang* deficiency by adding warm herbs like *Gui Zhi* (cinnamon) and *Fu Zi*. If in addition the physician wishes to boost the patient's *qi* level, he could choose to add some *Huang Qi* (astragalus) and *Xi Yang Shen* (American ginseng).

As each standard prescription is targeted at a particular syndrome, patients with several syndromes could have several standard prescriptions combined into one, with suitable adjustments to avoid duplication of herbs that are used in common by the different prescriptions, as well as modifications that reflect which syndrome the physician is treating as the priority, with larger amounts of the ingredients aimed at that syndrome, and which other syndromes he is treating more gently, with smaller quantities of the relevant herbs. Thus, the formulation of a prescription for a particular patient at a given time requires judgement and experience and, in a sense, is both a science and an art, much like the culinary recipes of an expert chef.

CHAPTER 4

CANCER PREVENTION AND TREATMENT USING TCM

TCM does not deal with cancer as a particular disease or a specific syndrome, and does not have a comprehensive theory explaining the origins of cancer and the principles of therapy for this family of diseases. Western medicine has postulated and discovered the causes of various kinds of cancer, tracing them to such factors as defective genes, environmental toxins, smoking, diet, stress and viruses. Modern oncology is a vast and complicated field, and TCM does not have theories and therapies that are equivalent to those offered by modern medicine.

The *Neijing* and other Chinese medical classics do describe conditions that are very similar to those found in cancer patients. For example, the *Neijing* describes in the *Suwen* "cough from the lungs, breathlessness and gasping, sometimes even with spitting out of blood... the pallor of the face indicating the reverse flow of *qi* (气逆)", a description of the telling symptoms of late-stage lung cancer. As to its cause, TCM attributes it to one or more syndromes: toxins in the lung (邪毒侵肺), accumulation of phlegm and dampness in the lung (痰湿内聚) and deficiency of healthy *qi* (正气内虚).

From the point of view of TCM theory, the formation of a cancerous tumour, its development and its eventual spread to other parts of the body has its origin in the loss of balance between *yin* and *yang* manifested in disorders involving the struggle between pathogens and healthy *qi*, and in excess and deficiency syndromes. Such disorders can be brought about by certain environmental and internal factors that predispose the body to them.

Combining knowledge from modern medicine with the perspectives of TCM, it has been possible to identify some of the principal factors that contribute to the incidence of cancers. Reducing exposure to or avoiding these predisposing factors can be regarded as ways of preventing or lowering the chances of contracting the disease.

We look next at some contributing factors commonly encountered in daily life that can be reduced or avoided.

4.1. Avoidance of Factors Contributing to Higher Incidence of Cancers

Based on estimates by the World Health Organization, about one third of cancers in the world can be prevented, another third can be cured and the last third can be treated to reduce suffering and prolong life.

The prevention of cancer can be approached on three fronts:

1. Avoidance and/or reduction of carcinogenic factors such as may be found in the environment (air pollution, water pollution, smoking, radiation exposure, etc) and in the diet (as in certain fermented foodstuffs, mouldy peanuts and the like).
2. Intervention in the interaction between carcinogenic factors and cells in the body to prevent the cells from turning cancerous.

3. Treating pre-cancerous growths and cellular changes to prevent them from developing into tumours; for example, removing polyps in the stomach and colon, or eliminating *Helicobacter pylori* colonies in the stomach lining that could develop into stomach cancers.

The first two approaches are the subject of much ongoing research, but current knowledge and resources do not enable us to consistently implement these preventive measures. However, pre-cancerous growths have been dealt with more successfully by modern diagnostic and treatment methods.

Drawing on TCM knowledge as well as modern medical experience, it may be useful to consider cancers as being caused by either internal or external factors, or a combination of the two. External factors constitute predisposing conditions for the development of tumours, whilst internal factors are decisive in determining if the body succumbs to external and internal causal factors. This viewpoint is consistent with the fact that all inhabitants in a given region and society are subject to about the same environmental influences, yet some contract cancers whilst others do not. This indicates that internal factors play the decisive role. Based on this approach, the following are some principal considerations for preventing the disease:

1. Eliminating or reducing external carcinogenic factors. This includes protecting employees at the workplace from harmful chemicals and pathogens and reducing environmental pollution. This is the responsibility of employers and government agencies, and is a critical factor in combating cancer. In addition, every individual should be vigilant against external carcinogenic factors and excessive radiation. For example, prolonged and intensive exposure to ultraviolet rays of the

sun can induce skin cancer. Many foodstuffs are also known or suspected to have carcinogens. These include smoked meats, barbecued foods, certain chemical fertilizers used to grow vegetables, and the consumption of foods lacking in trace elements iodine, selenium and molybdenum.

2. Some individuals have predisposing genetic factors. Where these have been discovered, appropriate steps to be taken could include increased vigilance to detect pre-cancerous growths and test for cancer markers. From the point of view of TCM, achieving internal *yin* and *yang* balance within the body is of paramount importance to reducing the possibility of succumbing to the disease. *Yin-yang* balance is achieved through time-honoured methods of health cultivation or *yangsheng*. These include changing unhealthy living habits such as smoking, eating food rich in fats and low in fibre and excessive alcohol consumption. It is also important to preserve internal emotional balance, avoiding anger, anxiety, sadness, fear and overindulgence in pleasures. Regular exercise and the practice of mind-calming exercises such as *taiji* and *qigong* are also very important. Certain herbal supplements are known to improve the body's internal defences (immune-system functions) against illness. These include herbs that tonify the spleen and kidney. Mushrooms, poria (*Fu Ling* 茯苓), *Zhu Ling* (猪苓), seaweed (海藻), astragalus (*Huang Qi* 黄芪), *Ling Zhi* (灵芝), *Nü Zhen Zi* (女贞子), *Xian Ling Pi* (仙灵脾) and *Gou Qi Zi* (枸杞子) are some of the more common herbs that are helpful in this respect.

3. Actively treat pre-cancerous growths or conditions that are potentially pre-cancerous. Examples of observable potential pre-cancerous growths and conditions include abnormalities on the skin and mucous membranes such as white spots on the mouth and throat mucous membranes, sores and ulcers

on the skin that do not heal after prolonged treatment, hyperplasia of the mammary gland, chronic ulcers and gastritis, ulcerative colorectitis, hepatitis B and C, liver cirrhosis, thickening of the lining of the cervix, and chronic inflammation of the pancreas.

4.2. Healthy Living for Cancer Prevention

A healthy lifestyle is the best way to ward off cancers. We suggest 15 living habits that could be helpful:

1. A balanced diet with adequate amounts of proteins, carbohydrates, fats, vitamins, minerals and fibre.
2. Avoid excessive food preferences and try not to eat the same food for prolonged periods. Have a change every so often.
3. Avoid excessive consumption of alcohol.
4. Avoid smoking as it harms both you and those around you.
5. Avoid too much salt in the food as salty food might predispose you to cancers.
6. Eat foodstuffs containing natural sources of vitamins A, C and E, and ensure you have sufficient fibre, fresh vegetables and whole grains in your diet.
7. Avoid overeating and becoming overweight.
8. Minimize the amount of fermented, smoked, fried and barbecued foods as these tend to have higher levels of carcinogens.
9. Avoid food that has turned rancid or gathered bacteria and fungi.
10. Avoid excessive exposure to the sun as ultraviolet rays can induce skin cancers.
11. Observe cleanliness and hygiene in daily habits, and avoid contact with substances that may or are known to contain

carcinogens (for example, certain PVC wrapping for food and building materials like asbestos). Stay away from public places that have been contaminated by chemical pollution.

12. Long working hours and fatigue can injure your immune system and predispose you to cancers.
13. Be careful to avoid emotional stress as this is harmful to the immune system and the body's defences against cancer. In TCM the seven harmful emotions are overindulgence in pleasure, anger, anxiety, grief, fear, shock and melancholy.
14. Regular exercise helps to strengthen the body against illnesses, including cancer.
15. Actively treat any symptoms that suggest pre-cancerous changes in the body.

The reader will note that about two thirds of these "prohibitions" have to do with diet; the importance of diet in cancer prevention cannot be overemphasized.

4.3. Principles of Using TCM in Cancer Treatment

Over my 40 years of clinical experience, I have observed that strengthening *qi* and improving blood circulation have important effects on the quality of life and prolonging life for cancer patients. Patients with late-stage cancers often have pronounced blood stasis problems; this is particularly so with lung cancers. I have also found that patients with stage 3 or stage 4 cancers have much higher rates of *qi* deficiency than those in stage 1 or 2. It is also apparent that chemotherapy can have severe effects on the body by inducing *qi* deficiency and blood stasis. Hence, strengthening *qi* and removing blood stasis using TCM herbs and acupuncture are important parts of the complementary arsenal for patients with late-stage cancers.

In general, illness in the human body has its origin in the loss of internal balance between *yin* and *yang*. From this point of view, cancerous growths have their fundamental origin in the loss of balance in several respects, for example between cancer cells and cells that suppress cancer growth, and between cell regeneration and cell division, resulting in rapid growth in the population of cancer cells. If we regard the factors that promote the growth of cancer cells and their spread as *yang* in character, and the suppression of cancerous tumours as *yin* in character, and also regard the increase in these factors as excess and their decline as deficiency, the entire picture fits into the TCM framework of viewing illness as reflecting several conditions: the struggle between healthy *qi* and pathogens, *yin-yang* imbalance and the presence of excess-deficiency syndromes (正邪阴阳虚实). It follows that the main treatment principle of cancer is to balance *yin* and *yang* and to strengthen the body's healthy *qi*; these in turn prevent the development of excess and deficiency syndromes.

For patients that have received treatment by surgery, chemotherapy or radiotherapy, some of these imbalances are in fact exacerbated by the treatment, resulting in a decline in the immune system, a weakening of the body to produce blood components like blood platelets, white blood cells and red blood cells, and the disruption of the digestive processes. This in turn causes a further weakening of *qi* and induces further imbalance. Hence, the holistic approach to managing cancer patients with complementary TCM therapy is to restore these imbalances, strengthen *qi* and remove blood stasis, regardless of the form of medical treatment the patient has undergone by Western medical methods for combating the tumour.

We discuss next specific complementary treatments for patients who have undergone each of the methods of Western treatment for tumours.

4.3.1. Patients who have undergone radiotherapy

Radiation therapy (radiotherapy) is used extensively in the treatment of cancers of the nasopharyngeal region, the upper oesophagus, throat, lung, cervix and uterus, and for mediastinal lymphoma. Radiotherapy basically can only achieve localized destruction of cancer cells and control their growth, but in the process it can also cause severe side effects for the whole body. The use of TCM herbs ameliorate the side effects and toxicities arising from this form of therapy besides consolidating the therapeutic effects of the treatment and prolonging the life span of the patient.

Within the TCM conceptual framework, the side effects of radiotherapy constitute a form of warm pathogen (热邪) that damages the body's *yin* and body fluids, compromises the digestive transforming function of the spleen and stomach, and inhibits the production of *qi*, resulting in various syndromes associated with these side effects. Patients who have undergone radiotherapy typically exhibit symptoms such as a dark tongue colour and pigmentation, suggesting blood stasis, as well as dry skin and dry throat; these in turn sometimes transform into internal heat.

TCM treatments for these syndromes include strengthening *qi* and nourishing *yin* (益气养阴), improving blood circulation and removing blood stasis (活血化瘀), regulating *qi* in the spleen and stomach, and tonification of the liver and kidney. Herbs commonly used for treating these syndromes are *Bei Sha Shen, Tai Zi Shen, Shi Hu, Yu Zhu, Tian Hua Fen, Ji Xue Teng, Nü Zhen Zi, Sheng Di, Xuan Shen, Ren Dong Teng, Wu Wei Zi, Shan Yao, Dang Gui, Jie Geng, Sheng Gan Cao, Sheng Huang Qi* and *Xi Yang Shen*. For treating blood stasis, the herbs commonly used are *Chuan Xiong, Hong Hua, Dan Shen* and *Ma Lin Zi*.

These herbs can also be used to enhance the effectiveness of radiotherapy.

4.3.2. Patients who have undergone chemotherapy

Chemotherapy is one of the most widely used form of treatment for cancer. Many new drugs enter the market each year, this being one of the most active areas of research for pharmaceutical companies in the West. As most patients who have undergone chemotherapy are well aware, one of the principal problems with chemotherapy is that it tends not to discriminate too well between the host body and the target adversary. In other words, in the process of combating cancer cells, much collateral damage is done to healthy cells in the body, particularly those with higher metabolic rates. Chemotherapy can induce nausea and vomiting, destruction of the bone marrow and the resultant reduction of blood cells, and a weakening of the immune system, hence lowering the body's defences against infection. Chemotherapy can damage the body's *yin* and the spleen-stomach digestive function and thereby affect liver and kidney functions as well as deplete the body's *qi* and blood. Consequently, patients undergoing chemotherapy often exhibit symptoms of giddiness, lassitude, low spirits, loss of appetite, insomnia or disturbed sleep, dry throat, and disturbance of bowel movements and urination.

It is in this area of chemotherapy side effects that I have found TCM to be able to contribute most to patient wellness, and one could say that this is one of the most successful areas of integrating Western and Chinese medicine.

In general, the best approach to treating chemotherapy side effects is strengthening the spleen and tonifying the kidney (健脾补肾). Among its principal benefits are the strengthening of the immune system and the restoration of the blood production function of the bone marrow, as well as the improvement in appetite and digestive function for nourishing the body.

The herbs used for the major side effects are as follows:

1. Increasing red blood cells: *Huang Qi* (黄芪), *Dang Shen* (党参), *Dang Gui* (当归), *Long Yan Rou* (龙眼肉), *Da Zao* (大枣), *Sheng Shu Di* (生熟地), *E Jiao* (阿胶), *Gui Ban Jiao* (龟板胶), *Lu Jiao Jiao* (鹿角胶), *Zi He Che* (紫河车), *Gou Qi Zi* (枸杞子) and *Ren Shen* (人参).

2. Increasing white blood cells: *Huang Qi* (黄芪), *Tai Zi Shen* (太子参), *Ren Shen* (人参), *Huang Jing* (黄精), *Nü Zhen Zi* (女贞子), *Tu Si Zi* (菟丝子), *Ji Xue Teng* (鸡血藤), *Zi He Che* (紫河车), *Dang Gui* (当归), *Hu Zhang* (虎杖), *Gang Ban Gui* (扛板归), *Shan Zhu Yu* (山茱萸), *Bu Gu Zhi* (补骨脂) and *Xian Ling Pi* (仙灵脾).

3. Increasing blood platelet count: *Nü Zhen Zi* (女贞子), *Han Lian Cao* (旱莲草), *Shan Zhu Yu* (山茱萸), *Sheng Di* (生地), *Da Zao* (大枣), *Sheng Huang Qi* (生黄芪), *Zi He Che* (紫河车), *Lu Jiao Jiao* (鹿角胶), *Bie Jia Jiao* (鳖甲胶), *Gui Ban Jiao* (龟板胶), *Ji Xue Teng* (鸡血藤), *Hua Sheng Yi* (花生衣), *Shi Wei* (石苇), *Chou Hu Lu* (抽葫芦), *Qian Cao Gen* (茜草根), *Sheng Ma* (升麻), *Gang Ban Gui* (扛板归) and *San Qi* (三七).

4. Strengthening the immune system: *Huang Qi* (黄芪), *Ren Shen* (人参), *Dang Shen* (党参), *Bai Zu* (白术), *Fu Ling* (茯苓), *Zhu Ling* (猪苓), *Ling Zhi* (灵芝), *Xiang Gu* (香菇), *Nü Zhen Zi* (女贞子), *Xian Ling Pi* (仙灵脾), *Gou Qi Zi* (枸杞子), *Tu Si Zi* (菟丝子) and *Bu Gu Zhi* (补骨脂).

4.3.3. Patients who have undergone surgery

Surgery remains the most common option for early-stage malignant tumours as it can be extremely effective and totally eliminate the disease. Every tumour is different; hence, each may require a slightly different surgical procedure. Certain post-surgery side effects in the body are commonly seen with cancer patients which TCM would characterize as "depletion of *qi* and damage to blood" (耗气伤血). This in turn causes disorders in the vital organs, meridians and *yin-yang* balance. Hence, before and after surgery, it would be appropriate to regulate the body to achieve a good state of balance, both to prepare the patient for the trauma of surgery and to help him recover from it.

4.3.3.1. *Pre-surgery care with TCM*

There are two aspects to preparing the patient for surgery.

The first is to strengthen the body's healthy *qi* using a variety of tonics suited to the person's constitution. These tonics combine one or both of two basic functions, fortifying the spleen and strengthening *qi* (健脾益气) and nourishing the liver and kidney (滋补肝肾). Among the well-known classical prescriptions used for these purposes are the Decoction of the Four Noble Herbs (四君子汤), *Bao Yuan Tang* (保元汤), *Ba Zhen Tang* (八珍汤) and *Shi Quan Da Bu Tang* (十全大补汤). These should be used after TCM diagnosis of the patient to determine his principal syndromes. In jurisdictions that allow it, intravenous injections of astragalus (*Huang Qi*) and ginseng (*Ren Shen*) can also be used to boost the body's healthy *qi*.

The second aspect of preparing the patient for surgery is to control the growth of the tumour before surgery using medicinal herbs, which some studies have found to achieve results similar to those of using a limited amount of chemotherapy before surgery. For example, some studies have found that the use of *Qiu Shui Xian Xian An* (秋水仙酰胺) before breast surgery to shrink the tumour and the use of *Ya Dan Zi* emulsion (鸭胆子乳剂) for stomach cancer can achieve better results than chemotherapy. However, in practice, surgery may be called for urgently and there may not be enough time for the relatively slow-acting Chinese herbs to achieve their objective. Hence, in general, preparing the patient for surgery using appropriate tonics is the more practical method.

4.3.3.2. *Post-surgery treatment*

My clinical experience with the care of cancer patients after surgery indicates that appropriate treatment with TCM herbs makes a significant difference to the patient's recovery and improves his chances of avoiding a relapse. I would recommend that the use of Chinese herbs begin as soon as the patient is able to consume food in the hospital. The method of post-surgery treatment would depend on the attending TCM physician in consultation with the surgeon and other doctors in charge of the patient. In practice, there are only a few principal methods from which to choose:

1. Regulating the functions of the spleen and stomach (调理脾胃). Owing to surgical trauma and the after-effects of anaesthesia, especially if surgery involves the alimentary canal, dysfunctioning of the digestive system is common, resulting sometimes in constipation, a bloated abdomen, loss of appetite, retention of wind in intestines, or a combination of these symptoms. Useful prescriptions include *Da Cheng Qi Tang* (大承气汤), *Xiao Cheng Qi Tang* (小承气汤) and *Xiang Sha Liu Jun Zi Tang* (香砂六君子汤).
2. Fortifying *qi* and consolidating the exterior (益气固表). Some patients suffer from excessive sweating owing to

weakness in the *qi* function of consolidating the exterior. The Jade Screen Decoction or *Yu Ping Feng San* (玉屏风散) is useful for this purpose. We can add *Wu Wei Zi* (五味子), *Hang Ju* (杭芍), *Fu Xiao Mai* (浮小麦), *Duan Long Gu* (煅龙骨) and *Duan Mu Li* (煅牡蛎) selectively, depending on the condition of the patient, to enhance the effects of this prescription for the individual patient.

3. Nourishing the *yin* and promoting clear fluids (养阴生津). Surgery often damages the *yin* and dries up the mucous membranes, causing symptoms such as a red tongue with little fur, dry mouth and throat, constipation (hardened faeces) and loss of appetite. Nourishing the *yin* and producing clear fluids is an appropriate approach to treatment. I once had a patient who had undergone surgery for colorectal cancer and suffered from such symptoms quite acutely. He had no appetite, lost a great deal of weight, had a red tongue with no fur and a deep, feeble and rapid pulse. After taking a prescription that contained a combination of *Sha Shen, Mai Dong, Shi Hu, Tian Hua Fen, Yu Zhu, Jie Geng, Zhu Ru, Sheng Di, Xuan Shen* and *Tai Zi Shen,* he recovered rapidly, regaining his appetite and his spirits. He did not follow up with chemotherapy but continued with Chinese medications. I last saw him eight years after surgery, and found him in a satisfactory state of health.

4.3.3.3. *Post-surgery treatment with TCM in the longer term*

It is not sufficient to cover only the immediate post-operative period for cancer patients. It is important that they follow up with appropriate tonics and other medications to achieve internal balance and an adequate level of healthy *qi*. This gives them a better chance to attain a better state of recovery as well as reducing the chances of a relapse. Two cases from my medical files are worthy of note. Case 1 was a patient who had his entire left lung and nearby lymph nodes removed because of lung cancer. After surgery he had an infection, high fever and adverse reaction to the intravenous drip. Recovery was very slow and he was too weak to get up from bed even three months after surgery. I intervened at this stage with TCM treatment, using the twin approach of combating pathogens and tonifying the body (攻补兼施). He gradually recovered, and the last time I saw him, seven years after surgery, his health was satisfactory. Case 2 was a Singaporean patient who had partial removal of the kidney because of a benign tumour in the kidney. Seven days after surgery, the drainage tube was not working satisfactorily and blood-like secretions were increasing in the drainage. The surgeon suggested a second operation to remove the whole kidney, but the patient was unwilling. I was requested through her friend to look into the matter, and decided to use Chinese herbs to treat her condition. I used the method of nourishing the liver and kidney, and also administered Yunnan white powder (云南白药) to treat her wound orally. Three days later, bleeding stopped, and seven days later the drainage tube was removed. We followed up with more TCM herbal treatment. Twenty years after the operation, I found her still fit and well.

4.4. Combining Western Medical and TCM Treatments

I have found from long experience of treating cancer patients that combining Western medical and TCM treatments generally yields the best results. In this regard, the four main principles to bear in mind are as follows:

1. The TCM approach of differentiating syndromes and applying therapy accordingly should be combined with identifying the disease by Western methods and treating the disease

specifically. For example, a patient with cancerous liver tumours should have these tumours reduced or eliminated by surgery and/or chemotherapy, but at the same time syndromes of spleen *qi* deficiency or blood stasis may be present as determined by TCM diagnosis. The latter should be treated with Chinese herbal medications.

2. It is necessary to treat the local disorder, such as a tumour or lesion, but also to examine imbalances in the body as a whole and treat the syndromes accordingly.

3. It may be necessary to combine the elimination of pathogens with the strengthening of the body with appropriate tonics. For example, a patient may have an excess syndrome of toxin accumulation and at the same time suffer from deficiency in *qi* or *yin*. The excess syndrome can be treated as a first priority but concurrently with gentle fortification of the body to mitigate the deficiency syndrome. When the excess syndrome has been eliminated, the treatment can then focus on the deficiency syndrome.

4. It is also necessary to consider short-term treatment and long-term therapy needs. The short-term need may be to eliminate heat pathogens or *qi* stagnation due to phlegm or dampness accumulation; the longer-term therapy may be that of building up the body's healthy *qi* to resist infections and improve motility in the digestive system and blood circulation.

In combining Western and Chinese therapies, we draw upon the best of each method of healing, using one to make up for inadequacies in the other and getting them to work together for greater therapeutic effect.

We conclude this chapter with a short discourse on the objective of medical treatment for cancer patients and its underlying ethical philosophy.

4.5. Preserving Life or Eliminating the Illness?

Many years ago, I visited a large hospital in Tianjin to see a patient with late-stage cancer with obvious symptoms of a rapid deterioration in condition. The attending Western medical doctor asked me if I had any special method for arresting the uncontrolled growth of his patient's tumour. I opined that his body was already very weak. In TCM terminology, he faced the prospect of a collapse and departure of his *yin* and *yang*, which portends imminent death, and any kind of aggressive destruction of the tumour was no longer appropriate. In such a situation, prolonging life and enhancing the quality of life was the main consideration rather than the elimination of the disease. Further radiotherapy or chemotherapy would only cause more suffering and likely shorten his life. The only choice available was that of boosting his healthy *qi* and immune system with a view to improving his quality of life, if not also his longevity.

CHAPTER 5

MAJOR FORMS OF CANCER AND CASE STUDIES

From the Medical Files of Professor Yu Rencun

Professor Yu Rencun has seen hundreds of cancer patients over many decades. These case studies have been chosen for illustrative purposes, indicating how TCM methods are combined with Western medical treatments to prolong and improve the quality of the lives of cancer patients and sometimes to bring about recovery. For each major form of cancer, two or three cases have been selected.

5.1. Lung Cancer

Lung cancer is the most common form of cancer and accounts for the largest number of deaths from cancer in developed countries. It is on the increase worldwide.

TCM associates one or more syndromes with lung cancer: toxins in the lung (邪毒侵肺), accumulation of phlegm and dampness in the lung (痰湿内聚) and deficiency of healthy *qi* (正气内虚), with the last syndrome as the dominating causal factor. Modern medicine attributes lung cancer to atmospheric pollution, smoking, harmful radiation and carcinogenic materials invading the body. However, as discussed in an earlier chapter, the cause of cancer is complex and is best viewed as a combination of many factors that predispose a person to the development and growth of cancerous tumours.

Western medicine treats lung cancer using one or more of three main methods, namely surgery, radiotherapy and chemotherapy. These treatments can be combined with TCM treatment, for which the patient is classified according to four major syndromes and complementary therapy administered accordingly. The four main syndromes are as follows:

1. *yin* deficiency with warm toxicity (阴虚毒热型);
2. phlegm and dampness accumulation (痰湿蕴肺);
3. blood stasis with toxicity (血瘀毒结型); and
4. deficiency of the lung and kidney (肺肾两虚型).

The following case studies illustrate how TCM is used in the treatment of a number of these syndromes.

Case 1

Male, 58 years old, ethnic han, married.

First visit: 6 September 1976
Main complaint: Chest pain, cough and sweating one week after exploratory thoracotomy for lung cancer.
History of present illness: Suffering from cough and discomforts like upper respiratory tract infection, the patient underwent fluoroscopy of the chest on 19 July 1976, which detected a shadow in the right lung. A chest X-ray on 25 July confirmed atelectasis of the middle lobe of his right lung. On the next day bronchofiberscope detection discovered granulation tissues at

the entrance of the right middle lobe and the biopsy and pathologic diagnosis indicated adenocarcinoma. An exploratory thoracotomy on the right side was performed on 31 August. Some metastatic lymph nodes with a firm texture existed on the right middle lobe and inferior porta pulmonis extending left into the mediastinum. Because of such a wide range of metastatic lymph nodes, from porta pulmonis to mediastinum, these could not be removed completely even if a complete pneumonectomy had been performed. The surgeons took a biopsy and located stainless marks on the surface of the lymph nodes in preparation for future radiotherapy; they did not proceed with further surgery to remove the tumour, and closed the thorax.

Past medical history: The patient suffered from stomach discomfort, abdominal distension and loose stools for over 20 years; hypotension, anaemia and dystrophia; susceptible to colds and lung infections. The patient had been smoking for 20 years and stopped in 1963. Since 1973, it was diagnosed as a complete right atrioventricular block.

Western medical diagnosis: Bronchial adenocarcinoma of the middle lobe of the right lung; metastatic lymph nodes from the right lung porta pulmonis to mediastinum; atelectasis of the middle lobe of the right lung.

Tongue and pulse manifestation: Pale tongue with tooth indentations and thin whitish fur; thin, slippery and slightly rapid pulse.

TCM differentiation of syndromes: Post-operational *qi* deficiency of the spleen and lung, masses of inner toxic phlegm.

Methods and principles of therapy: Replenishing *qi* and strengthening the exterior, reducing phlegm and resolving masses.

Prescription: Raw *Huang Qi* 30 g, parched *Bai Zhu* 10 g, *Fang Feng* 10 g, *Fu Xiao Mai* 30 g, calcined *Long Gu* 30 g, calcined *Mu Li* 30 g, prepared *Qian Hu* 12 g, *Ma Dou Ling* 10 g, raw *Pi Pa Ye* 10 g, *Cao He Che* 30 g, *Xia Ku Cao* 15 g, Sichuan *Bei Mu* 10 g, northern *Sha Shen* 15 g and *Wu Wei Zi* 10 g (six doses prescribed).

Second visit: 13 September 1976
After the patient took the last TCM prescription, symptoms of coughing and sweating were under control with less phlegm and good appetite. The tongue and pulse manifestation was unchanged. The method of therapy was maintained with the following modifications: eliminated *Pi Pa Ye* from the prescription and added *Zi Yuan* 12 g, *Ban Zhi Lian* 30 g and *Bai Hua She She Cao* 30 g.

Fourth visit: 27 September 1976
The patient had undergone radiotherapy seven times each with 200 cGy. His appetite had declined but cough was still under control. The tongue was pale red with tooth indentations while the pulse was still thin and slippery. To deal with the side effects of radiotherapy, TCM treatment shifted focus to tonifying the spleen and kidney, reducing phlegm and resolving tumour.
Prescription: Raw *Huang Qi* 30 g, *Dang Shen* 15 g, *Bai Zhu* 10 g, Yunnan *Fu Ling* 12 g, *Shen Qu* 10 g, *Tian Dong* 15 g, *Nü Zhen Zi* 15 g, *Tu Si Zi* 10 g, *Ji Xue Teng* 30 g, *Bei Mu* 10 g, *Qian Hu* 12 g, *Xia Ku Cao* 15 g, *Shi Wei* 30 g and *Ban Zhi Lian* 30 g.

Seventh visit: 18 October 1976
While undergoing radiotherapy, the patient had warm palms and frequent night urination. His bowel movements returned to normal. The tongue was still pale red and with tooth indentations. The pulse was thin, slippery and rapid.

Prescription: Removed *Tian Dong, Shen Qu, Qian Hu, Xia Ku Cao* and *Shi Wei* in the previous prescription and added *Sha Shen* 15 g, raw *Di Huang* 10 g, prepared *Di Huang* 10 g, *Dan Shen* 15 g, *Qian Shi* 12 g, *Ye Jiao Teng* 30 g and *Yi Zhi Ren* 12 g.

Subsequent visit: 15 November 1976
Radiotherapy treatment was completed without pronounced side effects, but the patient suffered from insomnia with warm palms. The tongue was pale red with tooth indentations and thin whitish fur. The left pulse was deep, thin and slippery; the right pulse was wiry and slippery. Considering that the radiotherapy had injured *yin* and depleted *qi*, TCM therapy was modified further to supplement *qi*, nourish *yin* and remove toxins to strengthen healthy *qi*.
Prescription: *Sha Shen* 30 g, raw *Di Huang* 10 g, prepared *Huang Qi* 30 g, *Ji Xue Teng* 30 g, *Nü Zhen Zi* 30 g, *Gou Qi Zi* 12 g, *Gua Lou* 30 g, *Bei Mu* 10 g, *Qian Hu* 12 g, *Tao Ren* 10 g, *Shan Dou Gen* 15 g, *Cao He Che* 30 g, *Long Kui* 30 g, *Ban Zhi Lian* 30 g and parched *Suan Zao Ren* 15 g.

20 December 1976 to April 1977
The patient had a cold and a fever accompanied by radiation pneumonia. The symptoms resolved after the administration of antibiotics and Chinese herbal medicines. The patient was given 5-fluorouridine chemotherapy 20 times totalling 20 g and CCNU 80 mg once. Meanwhile, TCM therapy was concurrently administered. The patient experienced only minimal side effects from chemotherapy.

Subsequent visit: 11 April 1977
Generally well, the patient was eating well and in good spirits. The tongue was still pale red with tooth indentations, the pulse thin, slippery and slightly fast. TCM treatment aimed to

consolidate the effects of tonifying the spleen and strengthening *qi*, removing toxins and resolving tumours.

Prescription: Raw *Huang Qi* 20 g, *Dang Shen* 15 g, *Bai Zhu* 10 g, raw *Shan Yao* 18 g, *Ban Xia* 12 g, *Sha Ren* 6 g, *Xia Ku Cao* 15 g, *Bei Mu* 10 g, *Hai Zao* 10 g, parched *Shan Zha* 10 g, parched *Shen Qu* 10 g, parched *Mai Ya* 10 g, *Sha Shen* 18 g, *Ban Zhi Lian* 30 g, *Bai Hua She She Cao* 30 g, *Long Kui* 30 g, *Qian Hu* 10 g and *Zi Wan* 10 g.

Since May 1977, the patient had been practising the New Guolin *qigong* therapeutic method, exercising four to five hours each day. His physical strength, appetite and spirits were much improved. The patient continued with Chinese medication for building resistance to dispel pathogenic factors. A chest X-ray review and comprehensive inspection each year found no recurrence of the tumour or metastasis. The patient went back to work early in 1979. ECG examination on 11 October 1979 found that the complete right bundle branch block was no longer present.

From 1980 to April 1983, his condition was stable. TCM therapy reverted to the original prescription with some modifications.

Prescription: Raw *Huang Qi* 30 g, *Dang Shen* 15 g, *Bai Zhu* 10 g, *Fu Ling* 10 g, parched *Shan Zha* 10 g, parched *Shen Qu* 10 g, parched *Mai Ya* 10 g, *Shan Yao* 10 g, parched *Jiang* 6 g, *Bai Ying* 30 g, *Long Kui* 30 g, *Nü Zhen Zi* 10 g, *Shou Wu Teng* 30 g, *Teng Li Gen* 30 g and *Shi Jian Chuan* 30 g.

From April 1983 to July 1984, he suffered occasionally from tachycardia and loose stools. The tongue was pale red and tooth-marked, with a thin whitish coating; the pulse was thready and slippery. The therapeutic principle remained basically the same: tonifying the spleen and supplementing *qi*, discharging toxins and resolving masses.

Prescription: Raw sun-dried *Ren Shen* 5 g (decocted separately), *Sha Shen* 30 g, *Tai Zi Shen* 20 g, raw *Huang Qi* 20 g, *Bai Zhu* 10 g, Yunnan *Fu Ling* 10 g, *Shan Yao* 10 g, parched *Shan Zha* 30 g, parched *Shen Qu* 30 g, parched *Mai Ya* 30 g, *Wu Wei Zi* 10 g, *Mai Dong* 15 g, Sichuan *Bei Mu* 10 g, *Xia Ku Cao* 15 g, *Bai Hua She She Cao* 15 g, wild *Ju Hua* 10 g and *Ma Wei Lian* 10 g.

From January 1985 to 1986, the patient continued to be treated for various ailments including tachycardia and diabetes with a combination of Western and Chinese medicines. Throughout this period the TCM approach of tonifying the spleen and strengthening *qi* remained a basic principle of treatment.

Last visit: 25 October 1986 (ten years and two months after cancer surgery)

The condition of the patient was stable. His appetite, urinary and bowel movements were normal, and diagnostic tests did not show anything significantly unusual. As a result, TCM herbal medical treatment was stopped.

The patient survived for another 13 years, finally succumbing to heart disease at the age of 81 and 23 years after surgery for lung cancer. Because of his courage in battling cancer and the success of the combined Western and TCM treatment that he received, he has been held up as a role model and was honoured for successfully combating and overcoming his illness.

Comments

In the past, some cancer patients resorted to treatment using only TCM because of the fear of surgery and the side effects of radiotherapy and chemotherapy. That was unfortunate because they deprived themselves of the opportunity to effectively treat their illnesses. In the 1970s when technology was less developed, surgery like exploratory thoracotomy done on the patient in Case 1 might have been needed to discover the complications of the growths in his thorax. But with modern technology such as CT scans, such exploratory surgery is no longer needed. This patient's case was one of advanced non-small cell cancer. What probably contributed to his recovery was the TCM medication that he received one week after surgery, which helped him to recover from surgery but also prepared him for the radiotherapy that followed.

Over the ten years of TCM treatment using herbal medications, I followed the principle on each examination of the patient of differentiating his syndromes as well as identifying any diseases present, and combined treatments for syndromes with those for diseases. We also combined anti-cancer cell treatment with promoting healthy *qi* in his body, as well as the treatment of local areas in the body with holistic healing. Promoting healthy *qi* was based mainly on fortifying the *qi* of his spleen and nourishing the kidney *yin*; combating cancer cells was based on clearing heat and removing toxins, softening and dispersing masses, resolving phlegm and dampness, eliminating blood stasis and reducing swellings.

After radiotherapy, the patient's immune system was weakened as evidenced by the main syndrome of the weakened spleen and kidney. This explained why the herbal prescriptions that he took contained a large component for strengthening *qi* and the kidney to boost his immune system and regulate the lung and spleen functions. The components for combating cancer cells took up only one quarter to one third of the prescription.

The patient also practised *qigong* which helped to balance *yin* and *yang* and promote circulation and build up the immune system. This complemented the herbal medications for building up his body's defences as well as for combating cancer cells. The patient thus received effective treatment of his condition on several fronts, and finally made a satisfactory recovery.

Case 2

Male, 71 years old, ethnic han, married.

First visit: 26 September 1997

Chief complaint: Operation for right lung cancer two years ago.

History of present illness: Pathologic report after operation in August 1995 showed adenocarcinoma, $T_1N_0M_0$. One cycle of chemotherapy began one week after the operation; no radiotherapy was administered. The patient also took TCM herbal decoctions for rehabilitation. Recently, he often suffered from cough with white sputum and chest pain. Urination and defecation appeared normal.

Past medical history: Hypertension for several years, controlled with drugs; relatively stable.

Tongue and pulse manifestation: Dark tongue with whitish coating. The pulse was taut and slippery.

Diagnosis of TCM: Lung masses.

Differentiation of syndromes: Deficiency of both *qi* and *yin*; accumulation of lung heat.

Methods and principles of therapy: Supplementing *qi* and nourishing *yin*; clearing away heat and toxic materials; dispersing phlegm and relieving cough.

Prescription: Raw *Huang Qi* 30 g, *Sha Shen* 30 g, *Mai Dong* 15 g, *Jie Geng* 10 g, *Qian Hu* 10 g, *Pi Pa Ye* 10 g, *Bai He* 10 g, *Long Kui* 10 g, *Bai Hua She She Cao* 20 g, *Cao He Che* 10 g, *Xing Ren* 10 g, Zhejiang *Bei Mu* 10 g, *Nü Zhen Zi* 15 g, *Gou Qi Zi* 10 g, Hangzhou *Bai Shao* 20 g, *Ji Nei Jin* 10 g and *Bai Bu* 10 g (one dose daily).

Subsequent visit: 6 February 1998
Frequent cough with white sputum. The tongue had a whitish coating while the pulse was deep, thready and fast. The same therapeutic approach as before was used with the following modifications: added *Wu Wei Zi* 6 g, *Sang Bai Pi* 10 g, *Yu Xing Cao* 30 g, *Bai Ying* 15 g and *She Mei* 15 g and removed *Jie Geng*, *Qian Hu*, *Pi Pa Ye*, *Bai Bu*, *Bai He*, *Cao He Che* and Hangzhou *Bai Shao*.

Subsequent visit: 3 September 1998
Cough with shortness of breath and white lumpy sputum. The tongue was dark red with petechiae while the root had yellow greasy fur. The pulse was thready, taut and slippery.
Prescription: *Fei Ji* capsules (肺积胶囊) and *Xian Cao* pills (仙草丹) and the following decoction: *Qian Hu* 10 g, *Xing Ren* 10 g, *Sha Shen* 30 g, *Tai Zi Shen* 30 g, *Mai Dong* 15 g, *Wu Wei Zi* 10 g, raw *Huang Qi* 30 g, *Bai Ying* 30 g, *Long Kui* 20 g, *Shi Jian Chuan* 15 g, *Cao He Che* 15 g, parched *Shan Zha* 10 g, parched *Shen Qu* 10 g, parched *Mai Ya* 10 g, *Ji Xue Teng* 30 g and *Gou Qi Zi* 10 g.

Subsequent visit: 25 December 1998
Dry mouth at night, cough with thick white sputum which was difficult to expectorate. Appetite was good but sleep poor; urination and defecation normal; the tongue dark red with petechiae, root yellowish. The pulse was thready and

taut. The syndrome was differentiated as deficiency of both *qi* and *yin*; heat toxicity and blood stasis. The methods and principles of therapy were supplementing *qi* and nourishing *yin*, detoxification and removing stasis.

Prescription: *Bai Ying* 30 g, *Long Kui* 20 g, *Bai Hua She She Cao* 30 g, *Shi Jian Chuan* 15 g, *Gui Jian Yu* 10 g, *Ji Xue Teng* 30 g, *Yu Xing Cao* 30 g, *Sha Ren* 10 g, *Ji Nei Jin* 10 g, *Sha Shen* 30 g, *Tai Zi Shen* 30 g, raw *Huang Qi* 30 g, *Mai Dong* 15 g and *Wu Wei Zi* 10 g.

Subsequent visit: 26 February 1999
The patient caught a cold and had a cough with white sputum, running nose and a dull ache in the upper part of the body. His appetite was good while sleep was poor. The stools were a little bit loose. The tongue was dark red with petechiae; its root had yellow-white greasy fur; the pulse was deep, taut and slippery. Modified *Er Chen* Decoction (二陈汤) was used to strengthen the spleen and harmonize the middle abdomen, detoxify and promote blood flow.

Prescription: *Bai Zhu* 10 g, *Chen Pi* 10 g, *Fu Ling* 10 g, *Ban Xia* 10 g, raw *Huang Qi* 30 g, *Tai Zi Shen* 30 g, parched *Shan Zha* 10 g, parched *Shen Qu* 10 g, parched *Mai Ya* 10 g, *Xing Ren* 10 g, raw *Yi Yi Ren* 15 g, *Ji Nei Jin* 10 g, *Bai Ying* 30 g, *Cao He Che* 15 g, *Dan Shen* 15 g, *Ji Xue Teng* 30 g and *Gou Qi Zi* 10 g.

Date of visit: 24 September 1999
The patient's condition was normal except for a bit of coughing and slightly elevated blood pressure. The tongue was dark red with petechiae; the root of it had a white coating. The pulse was deep and taut. The method of therapy was modified to supplementing *qi* and tonifying the kidney; detoxicating and activating blood flow.

Prescription: Raw *Huang Qi* 30 g, *Dan Shen* 15 g, *Ji Xue Teng* 30 g, *Chi Shao* 15 g, *Chuan Xiong* 15 g, *Nü Zhen Zi* 15 g, *Gou Qi Zi* 10 g, *Tai Zi Shen* 30 g, *Du Zhong* 10 g, *Tian Ma* 10 g, *Bai Ying* 30 g, *Long Kui* 20 g, *Bai Hua She She Cao* 30 g, *Sha Ren* 10 g, parched *Shan Zha* 10 g, parched *Shen Qu* 10 g and parched *Mai Ya* 10 g.

Subsequent visit: 28 January 2000
Dry mouth and nose, cough with much sputum. The tongue was dark red with petechiae and a thin white coating. The pulse was thin, slippery and string-like.
Prescription: *Qian Hu* 10 g, *Xing Ren* 10 g, *Zi Wan* 10 g, *Bai Zhu* 10 g, *Sha Shen* 30 g, *Mai Dong* 15 g, *Ji Xue Teng* 30 g, raw *Huang Qi* 30 g, *Bai Ying* 30 g, *Long Kui* 15 g, *Cao He Che* 15 g, *Bai Hua She She Cao* 30 g, parched *Shan Zha* 10 g, parched *Shen Qu* 10 g, parched *Mai Ya* 10 g, *Sha Ren* 10 g and *Zhi Qiao* 10 g. Continued with *Fei Ji* capsules and *Xian Cao* pills.

Subsequent visit: 9 August 2002
More than six years after the operation for right upper lobe cancer, the sputum was white and sticky with less coughing; appetite, urination and defecation were normal; the tongue was pale and darkish with a thin whitish coating; the pulse was thready and slippery.
Prescription: *Qian Hu* 10 g, *Xing Ren* 10 g, *Sha Shen* 30 g, Sichuan *Bei Mu* 10 g, raw *Huang Qi* 30 g, *Tai Zi Shen* 30 g, *Dan Shen* 15 g, *Chuan Xiong* 15 g, *Bai Hua She She Cao* 30 g, *Bai Ying* 30 g, *Long Kui* 20 g, *She Mei* 15 g, parched *Shan Zha* 10 g, parched *Shen Qu* 10 g, parched *Mai Ya* 10 g, *Ji Nei Jin* 10 g, *Sha Ren* 10 g and *Cao He Che* 15 g.

Subsequent visit: 30 January 2004
More than eight years after surgery, the patient had no coughing but there was a bit of sputum. The tongue was dark red

with petechiae and a white coating. The pulse was deep, thready and taut.

Prescription: Raw *Huang Qi* 30 g, *Tai Zi Shen* 30 g, *Mai Dong* 15 g, *Wu Wei Zi* 10 g, *Xing Ren* 10 g, Sichuan *Bei Mu* 10 g, *Cao He Che* 15 g, *Shi Shang Bai* 15 g, *Sha Shen* 30 g, *Dan Shen* 15 g, parched *Shan Zha* 10 g, parched *Shen Qu* 10 g, parched *Mai Ya* 10 g, *Ji Xue Teng* 30 g, *Ji Nei Jin* 10 g, *Sha Ren* 10 g, *Nü Zhen Zi* 15 g and *Gou Qi Zi* 10 g.

Subsequent visit: 2 April 2004

The patient had an infection on his left foot for the recent two weeks which was resolved after treatment. He had a good appetite but poor sleep; dry stools and frequent urination at night. The tongue was dark red with petechiae and a white coating; the pulse was deep, thready and taut.

Prescription: *Sha Shen* 30 g, *Mai Dong* 15 g, *Tai Zi Shen* 30 g, raw *Huang Qi* 30 g, *Shan Yu Rou* 10 g, *Fu Pen Zi* 10 g, *Gou Qi Zi* 10 g, *Nü Zhen Zi* 15 g, *Dan Shen* 15 g, *Ji Xue Teng* 30 g, *Bai Ying* 30 g, *Ban Zhi Lian* 15 g, parched *Shan Zha* 10 g, parched *Shen Qu* 10 g, parched *Mai Ya* 10 g, *Sha Ren* 10 g and Sichuan *Bei Mu* 10 g. Continued with *Fei Ji* capsules.

From then on, the patient insisted on TCM rehabilitation. The core combination of the prescription was similar to the previous one. With ageing, some geriatric symptoms emerged, such as fluctuation of blood pressure (a little above the normal level sometimes) and frequent urination. These symptoms were due to the deficiency of kidney *qi*. The tongue was dark red with petechiae. The following prescription was used since July 2004: *Tai Zi Shen* 30 g, *Mai Dong* 15 g, *Wu Wei Zi* 10 g, *Sha Shen* 30 g, raw *Huang Qi* 30 g, *Dan Shen* 15 g, *Ji Xue Teng* 30 g, *Nü Zhen Zi* 15 g, *Gou Qi Zi* 10 g, *Shan Yu Rou* 10 g, *Tu Si Zi* 10 g, *Fu Pen*

Zi 10 g, parched *Shan Zha* 10 g, parched *Shen Qu* 10 g, parched *Mai Ya* 10 g, *Ji Nei Jin* 10 g, *Sha Ren* 10 g and Zhejiang *Bei Mu* 10 g.

The next visit took place in January 2006. The patient continued with the TCM herbal decoction with three doses per week. The principle remained that of supplementing *qi* and tonifying the kidney; detoxicating and activating blood flow. More than ten years had passed since the operation was carried out. He was fine and in good spirits, and had a good appetite. Although in his eighties, he still participated in work and social activities.

Comments

This patient had early-stage lung cancer, in principle not requiring post-operative Western medical treatment. However, the patient insisted on using TCM for rehabilitation after surgery, with a view to preventing a recurrence of the illness and improving his life quality. During the period of therapy, the herbal prescription was modified according to the syndromes and with the purpose of prevention. The methods and principles of therapy — supplementing *qi* and tonifying the kidney, detoxicating and activating blood flow — could also delay ageing and prevent premature senility, and the patient was committed to maintaining this kind of health therapy. Apart from the daily decoctions, *Fei Ji* capsules were used to strengthen healthy *qi* and resist cancer, and *Xian Cao* pills (made by the Beijing Hospital of TCM) to supplement *qi* and consolidate the kidney for better body resistance. The patient's chance of survival was enhanced and his life span increased.

Case 3

Female, 46 years old, ethnic han, married.

First visit: 1 June 2004

Chief complaint: Lesion in right lung discovered four months ago; brain metastasis. Western medical diagnosis: Right lung adenocarcinoma with brain metastasis.

History of present illness: The patient experienced breathing difficulties. CT scan in January 2004 found a space-occupying lesion in the right lung, with brain metastasis. Bronchoscopy showed medium-low differentiated adenocarcinoma. Brain radiotherapy was administered 20 times, with the total dose reaching 4000 cGy. The drug Iressa was used for nearly three months from February 2004. CT scan showed that the lesion diminished by April.

Present symptoms: The symptoms were alleviated after radiotherapy and chemotherapy. The patient felt fullness at the middle and upper parts of the oesophagus and difficulty in expectoration; had dryness of the throat; was not eating and sleeping well; and had normal bowel and urinary functions. There was a mild delay in menstruation.

Past medical history: No chronic disease or infectious disease.

TCM diagnosis: Dark red tongue with white thin fur; deep, thready and taut pulse.

Syndrome differentiation: Qi and *yin* deficiency with phlegm and accumulation of toxins.

Method of treatment: Replenishing *qi* and nourishing *yin*, clearing phlegm and toxins.

Prescription: Sha Shen 30 g, Mai Dong 15 g, Wu Wei Zi 10 g, Tai Zi Shen 30 g, Tian Hua Fen 15 g, Gou Qi Zi 10 g, Nü Zhen Zi 15 g, Dan Pi 12 g, Ji Xue Teng 30 g, Bai Xian Pi 10 g, Shan Yu

Rou 10 g, *Jie Geng* 10 g, raw *Gan Cao* 6 g, fried *Zao Ren* 20 g, charred *Shan Zha* 10 g, charred *Mai Ya* 10 g, charred *Shen Qu* 10 g, *Sha Ren* 10 g and *Quan Xie* 3 g.

Second visit: 4 September 2004
Present condition: The patient had a sore throat, with a little white phlegm; was eating and sleeping well; had normal bowel movements and urination; and had a dark tongue with white thin fur and a deep, thready and weak pulse.
Prescription: *Fu Ling* 10 g, *Bai Zhu* 10 g, *Sha Shen* 30 g, raw *Huang Qi* 30 g, *Tai Zi Shen* 30 g, *Gou Qi Zi* 10 g, *Nü Zhen Zi* 15 g, *Sha Ren* 10 g, *Shan Yu Rou* 10 g, *Dan Pi* 12 g, *Bai Xian Pi* 12 g, *Che Qian Cao* 15 g, *Cao He Che* 15 g, *Mai Dong* 15 g, charred *Shan Zha* 10 g, charred *Mai Ya* 10 g, charred *Shen Qu* 10 g and *Ji Nei Jin* 10 g.

Third visit: 19 October 2004
Present condition: The patient had itchy skin, sore throat, irregular menstruation for the last two to three months, fatigue and no coughing. She was sleeping well, had normal bowel movements and urination, and mouth ulcers. The tongue was dark with petechiae and white fur; the pulse was deep, thready and weak.
Prescription: *Sha Shen* 30 g, *Shu Di* 12 g, *Shan Yu Rou* 10 g, *Shan Yao* 10 g, *Fu Ling* 10 g, *Dan Pi* 12 g, *Ze Xie* 10 g, fried *Zhi Mu* 10 g, fried *Huang Bai* 10 g, *Bai Xian Pi* 10 g, raw *Huang Qi* 30 g, *Tai Zi Shen* 30 g, *Ji Xue Teng* 30 g, *Cao He Che* 15 g, charred *Shan Zha* 10 g, charred *Mai Ya* 10 g, charred *Shen Qu* 10 g, *Ji Nei Jin* 10 g and *Sha Ren* 10 g.

Fourth visit: 7 December 2004
Present condition: The patient's diarrhoea and skin eczema were improving; her menses stopped for three months; she had no coughing, occasional oral ulcers, and was thirsty

especially at night. She was eating well, with normal bowel movements. The tongue was dark red with white thin fur; the pulse was deep and thready.

Prescription: *Sha Shen* 30 g, *Mai Dong* 15 g, *Bai Xian Pi* 10 g, raw *Huang Qi* 30 g, *Tai Zi Shen* 30 g, *Fu Ling* 10 g, *Bai Zhu* 10 g, *Gou Qi Zi* 10 g, *Nü Zhen Zi* 15 g, *Shan Yu Rou* 10 g, *Xia Ku Cao* 15 g, *Zhe Bei* 10 g, charred *Shan Zha* 10 g, charred *Mai Ya* 10 g, charred *Shen Qu* 10 g, *Ji Nei Jin* 10 g, *Sha Ren* 10 g, *Wu Gong* 1 piece, *Jie Geng* 10 g and raw *Gan Cao* 6 g.

Fifth visit: 11 January 2005
Present condition: The ALT a little higher than the normal level; regular menstruation returned after taking the herbal medicine. The patient was eating and sleeping well, with normal bowel movements and urination. The tongue was dark red with thin white fur; the pulse was deep and thready.

Prescription: *Yin Chen* 10 g, *Jiang Huang* 10 g, *Fu Ling* 10 g, *Bai Zhu* 10 g, *Sha Shen* 30 g, raw *Huang Qi* 30 g, *Tai Zi Shen* 30 g, *Gou Qi Zi* 10 g, *Nü Zhen Zi* 15 g, *Ji Xue Teng* 30 g, *Jie Geng* 10 g, *Zhe Bei* 10 g, charred *Shan Zha* 10 g, charred *Mai Ya* 10 g, charred *Shen Qu* 10 g, *Ji Nei Jin* 10 g, *Sha Ren* 10 g, *Wu Gong* 1 piece and *Zhu Ru* 10 g.

Sixth visit: 23 February 2005
Present condition: The patient had dry itchy skin; she was eating and sleeping well, with normal bowel movements and urination, and normal menstruation. The tongue was dark with thin white fur; the pulse was deep, thready and weak.

Prescription: *Yin Chen* 15 g, *Jiang Huang* 12 g, *Fu Ling* 10 g, *Bai Zhu* 10 g, raw *Huang Qi* 30 g, *Tai Zi Shen* 30 g, *Gou Qi Zi* 10 g, *Nü Zhen Zi* 15 g, *Bai Xian Pi* 10 g, *Dan Pi* 12 g, *Zhe Bei* 10 g, *Sha Shen* 30 g, *Chi Shao* 10 g, *Ju Hong* 10 g, *Xing Ren* 10 g, charred *Shan Zha* 10 g, charred *Mai Ya* 10 g, charred *Shen Qu* 10 g, *Ji Nei Jin* 10 g, *Sha Ren* 10 g, *Di Fu Zi* 10 g and fried *Gan Cao* 6 g.

Seventh visit: 12 April 2005
Present condition: The patient was in stable condition; her skin was less dry and itchy; she had a little rash on the face and nose. She was eating and sleeping well, with a tendency for diarrhoea after eating raw and cold foods; she had normal bowel movements and urination, and normal menstruation. The tongue was dark with white thin fur; the pulse was deep, thready and weak.
Prescription: *Yin Chen* 15 g, *Jiang Huang* 12 g, *Tu Fu Ling* 10 g, *Bai Zhu* 10 g, raw *Huang Qi* 30 g, *Tai Zi Shen* 30 g, *Gou Qi Zi* 10 g, *Nü Zhen Zi* 15 g, *Bai Xian Pi* 10 g, *Zhe Bei* 10 g, *Shan Yu Rou* 10 g, *Cao He Che* 15 g, charred *Shan Zha* 10 g, charred *Mai Ya* 10 g, charred *Shen Qu* 10 g, *Chen Pi* 10 g, *Ban Xia* 9 g, *Ji Nei Jin* 10 g, *Sha Ren* 10 g, *Di Fu Zi* 10 g and fried *Gan Cao* 6 g.

Eighth visit: 22 June 2006
Present condition: The patient was eating and sleeping well, with an aversion to greasy food and some loss of taste. The tongue was dark with petechiae and white thin fur; the pulse was deep and thready.
Prescription: *Sha Shen* 30 g, *Tai Zi Shen* 30 g, raw *Huang Qi* 30 g, *Mai Dong* 15 g, *Wu Wei Zi* 10 g, *Gou Qi Zi* 10 g, *Nü Zhen Zi* 15 g, *Xian Ling Pi* 10 g, *Shan Yu Rou* 10 g, *Bai Zhu* 10 g, *Fu Ling* 10 g, *Zhi Qiao* 10 g, charred *Shan Zha* 10 g, charred *Mai Ya* 10 g, charred *Shen Qu* 10 g, *Ji Nei Jin* 10 g, *Sha Ren* 10 g, *Cao He Che* 15 g, fried *Zao Ren* 20 g and *Shou Wu Teng* 30 g.

Ninth visit: 13 July 2006
Present condition: Similar to eighth visit, with some loose stools.

Prescription: *Tai Zi Shen* 30 g, raw *Huang Qi* 30 g, *Bai Zhu* 10 g, *Fu Ling* 10 g, *Zhi Qiao* 10 g, *Gou Qi Zi* 10 g, *Nü Zhen Zi* 15 g, *Xian Ling Pi* 10 g, *Shan Yu Rou* 10 g, *Bai Xian Pi* 10 g, *Sha Shen* 30 g, fried *Zao Ren* 20 g, *Shou Wu Teng* 30 g, charred *Shan Zha* 10 g, charred *Mai Ya* 10 g, charred *Shen Qu* 10 g, *Ji Nei Jin* 10 g, *Sha Ren* 10 g, *Jie Geng* 10 g and raw *Gan Cao* 6 g.

Comments

This is a case of lung adenocarcinoma with brain metastasis, classified as non-small cell lung cancer. The patient received only palliative brain radiotherapy with no chemotherapy. Only the drug Iressa and Chinese herbal medicine were used, and this stabilized the patient's condition. Iressa is effective in the treatment of non-small cell lung cancer, with possible side effects of diarrhoea and skin rash, which Chinese herbal medicine can help alleviate. The patient was diagnosed as having *qi* and *yin* deficiency with phlegm and toxin aggregation. *Sha Shen, Mai Dong, Tai Zi Shen, Bai Zhu*, raw *Huang Qi, Fu Ling, Wu Wei Zi, Gou Qi Zi, Nü Zhen Zi, Tian Hua Fen* and *Shan Yu Rou* can replenish *qi*, nourish *yin* and strengthen healthy *qi*; *Xia Ku Cao, Bei Mu, Jie Geng* and *Cao He Che* can remove phlegm and masses; *Ji Xue Teng* can promote blood circulation and remove obstruction in channels; *Quan Xie* and *Wu Gong* can calm wind and relieve convulsions and are especially good for brain metastasis; and *Dan Pi, Bai Xian Pi* and *Di Fu Zi* can cool blood and clear the skin to deal with the side effects of Iressa on skin, which helped the patient to survive for more than two years after brain metastasis.

5.2. Breast Cancer

In breast cancer the endothelial cells of the lacteal gland duct lose their normal character and become incapable of self-repair. The main clinical manifestation is a lacteal gland tumour. Breast cancer tumours generally tend to develop slowly.

Breast cancer is among the most commonly occurring form of malignant tumour in women. Its incidence and mortality rate vary widely across different regions in the world, and historically have been higher in Europe and America than in Africa, Latin America and Asia.

In China, the incidence of breast cancer in the cities is increasing rapidly and approaching the Western rate, being higher in Shanghai, Beijing and Tianjin, with Shanghai topping the list. Research has shown that this increasing incidence of breast cancer is related to higher incomes and an increase in the intake of foods high in fats, later age at first pregnancy and the declining practice of breast-feeding.

The Chinese medical classics mentioned breast cancer from early historical times. In AD 610, Chao Yuanfang of the Sui dynasty mentioned *shiyong* (石痈) in his *Treatise on the Pathogenesis and Manifestations of All Diseases*, describing it as a tumour that "can be felt definitely, with a root. The core and the surface are closely bonded, with slight pain but without heat. It is as hard as a stone". In the Song dynasty, Chen Ziming discussed the differences between *ruyong* (breast carbuncle) and *ruyan* (breast tumour) in *The Compendium of Effective Prescriptions for Women* (AD 1237). In the Yuan dynasty, Zhu Danxi mentioned in *Gezhi yulun* (*An Inquiry into the Properties of Things*) (1347) that "the accumulation of depression or anger consumes spleen *qi*, and thus liver *qi* cannot be controlled and is reversed upward to form a tumour like a big chess piece, without pain or itching".

On the aetiology and pathogenesis of breast cancer, classical Chinese medical literature differentiates between external and internal factors. On external factors, the *Treatise on the Pathogenesis and Manifestations of All Diseases* mentions that the disease "happens in patients with weak constitutions attacked by the pathogens of wind and cold, leading to blood stasis". As for internal factors, much of the classical literature cites emotional factors, specifically liver depression with *qi* stagnation harming the spleen, leading to disorders of *qi* and blood circulation and of the *zang-fu* organ functions. The disease was also observed to occur mainly among middle-aged women with depression or accumulated anger (Yu Bo, *Orthodox Manual of Medicine*). This is consistent with the statistics on breast cancer gathered from Western clinical records indicating emotional factors as an underlying cause of the disease.

5.2.1. Treatment of breast cancer

The treatment plan for breast cancer should be in accordance with the clinical stage of the disease, TCM differentiation of syndromes, and the patient's constitution. Combining radiotherapy, chemotherapy and endocrine therapy with TCM treatment often gets the best results for prolonging and improving the quality of life of the patient.

After surgery for breast cancer, the main TCM syndrome manifestations are *qi* and blood deficiency and imbalances in the spleen and stomach. TCM treatment should be applied to replenish *qi* and nourish blood, and to regulate the spleen and stomach. Herbs such as *Sheng Huang Qi, Tai Zi Shen, Ji Xue Teng, Bai Zhu, Fu Ling, Ji Nei Jin, Sha Ren* and *Mu Xiang* can be used.

Patients during chemotherapy may experience fatigue, nausea, poor appetite and low white blood cell count; the tongue is pale red or slightly dark, with thin white or yellowish fur; the pulse is thready and rapid or taut. For patients with *qi* deficiency and blood stasis and spleen and kidney deficiency, we should replenish *qi* and activate blood, replenish the spleen and tonify the kidney. *Sheng Xue Tang Jia Wei* (Modified *Sheng Xue Decoction*) (生血汤加味) can be applied. The specific drugs used are as follows: raw *Huang Qi* 30 g, *Tai Zi Shen* 30 g, *Bai Zhu* 10 g, *Fu Ling* 10 g, *Nü Zhen Zi* 10 g, *Gou Qi Zi* 10 g, *Sheng Shan Yao* 15 g, *Ju Pi* 10 g, *Zhu Ru* 10 g, *Ji Nei Jin* 10 g, *Jiao San Xian* 10 g each, *Ji Xue Teng* 30 g and *Zhi Gan Cao* 6 g. In this formulation, *Huang Qi*, *Tai Zi Shen*, *Bai Zhu*, *Fu Ling* and *Zhi Gan Cao* can replenish the spleen and tonify *qi*; *Ji Xue Teng* can promote blood circulation; *Ju Pi* and *Zhu Ru* can alleviate nausea; *Nü Zhen Zi*, *Gou Qi Zi* and *Sheng Shan Yao* tonify the kidney; and *Ji Nei Jin* and *Jiao San Xian* improve the appetite.

Variations on the prescription: add *Ban Xia* 10 g to stop nausea; add *Zi He Che* 10 g if there is anaemia or weakening of the blood functions; add *Qian Cao* 15 g and 6 pieces of *Da Zao* when blood platelet count is low; add *Xian Ling Pi* 10 g when the immune function is weakened.

Patients during radiotherapy may suffer from lassitude, dryness and bitterness in the mouth, poor appetite, and reduced white blood cell count. The tongue is dark or purple with thin or no fur; the pulse is thready and rapid or thready and wiry. These are symptoms of *qi* and *yin* deficiency. We should replenish *qi* and nourish *yin* and apply the following herbs: *Bei Sha Shen* 30 g, *Mai Dong* 15 g, *Shi Hu* 10 g, *Sheng Huang Qi* 30 g, *Tai Zi Shen* 30 g, *Bai Zhu* 10 g, *Fu Ling* 10 g, *Dang Gui* 10 g, *Nü Zhen Zi* 10 g, *Gou Qi Zi* 10 g, *Sheng Shan Yao* 15 g, *Ji Nei Jin* 10 g, *Jiao San Xian* 10 g each, *Ji Xue Teng* 30 g and *Zhi Gan Cao* 6 g.

Bei Sha Shen, *Mai Dong* and *Shi Hu* nourish *yin*; *Dang Gui* nourishes the blood; *Sheng Huang Qi*, *Tai Zi Shen*, *Bai Zhu*, *Fu*

Ling and *Zhi Gan Cao* strengthen the spleen and tonify *qi*; *Ji Xue Teng* promotes blood circulation; *Nü Zhen Zi*, *Gou Qi Zi* and *Sheng Shan Yao* tonify the kidney; and *Ji Nei Jin* and *Jiao San Xian* promote digestion. If skin problems appear during radiotherapy, external medicine *Hei Jiang Dan* formulated by the Beijing Hospital of TCM may be used.

The main TCM syndromes seen in breast cancer patients are liver depression with *qi* stagnation, *chong* meridian and *ren* meridian disorder (冲任经络失调) and the accumulation of heat toxins.

For liver depression with *qi* stagnation, a condition often related to emotional stress, the patient feels swelling and pain in the breasts and sides of the thorax, irritability, a bitter taste in the mouth, dry throat, dizziness and blurred vision; the tongue fur is thin and white or yellowish; the pulse is taut and slippery. These indicate stagnation of liver *qi* and phlegm coagulation. The therapeutic approach for such a condition is soothing the liver and regulating *qi*, dissipating phlegm and dispersing accumulations. A suitable prescription comprises *Chai Hu* 10 g, *Qing Pi* 10 g, *Yu Jin* 10 g, *Ju Ye* 10 g, *Dang Gui* 10 g, *Bai Shao* 10 g, *Yun Ling* 10 g, *Gua Lou* 30 g, *Bai Zhu* 10 g, *Shan Ci Gu* 15 g, *Bai Zhi* 10 g.

Because the breasts are located in the chest through which the liver meridian passes, when the liver fails in its basic function to facilitate *qi* flow, symptoms appear in the form of distension and pain in the breasts and sides of the thorax, characteristic of liver depression. Liver depression with spleen deficiency causes phlegm and turbid *qi* accumulation in the body with *qi* stagnation and blood stasis in the breasts. *Chai Hu*, *Qing Pi*, *Yu Jin* and *Ju Ye* soothe the liver and regulate *qi*; *Dang Gui* and *Bai Shao* nourish the blood and liver; *Gua Lou*, *Shan Ci Gu* and *Bai Zhi* dissipate phlegm and disperse accumulations; and *Yun Ling* and *Bai Zhu* strengthen the spleen and remove dampness.

In the case of *chong* and *ren* meridian disorders, the main symptoms are those for liver *qi* stagnation enumerated earlier, but there is also the possibility of irregular menstruation, soreness and weakness in the lower back and knee, a feverish sensation in the palms of the hands, soles of the feet and chest, irritation in the eyes and a dry mouth. The therapeutic approach is to regulate the two meridians, and nourish the liver and kidney. A suitable prescription would comprise the following: *Xiang Fu* 10 g, *Yu Jin* 10 g, *Chuan Lian Zi* 10 g, *Dang Gui* 12 g, *Sheng Shu Di* 15 g each, *Bai Shao* 15 g, *Chuan Xiong* 10 g, *Ju Ye* 10 g, *Nü Zhen Zi* 10 g, *Gou Qi Zi* 15 g, *Sheng Shan Yao* 15 g, *Ye Ju Hua* 15 g and *Gua Lou* 30 g.

Liver depression transforms stagnant *qi* into fire, which consumes body fluids and causes liver and kidney *yin* deficiency, which in turn leads to the disorder of the *chong* and *ren* meridians. *Dang Gui, Sheng Shu Di, Bai Shao, Chuan Xiong, Nü Zhen Zi* and *Gou Qi Zi* nourish *yin* and blood, tonify the kidney and regulate menstruation; *Xiang Fu, Yu Jin, Chuan Lian Zi* and *Ju Ye* soothe the liver and regulate *qi*; *Sheng Shan Yao* replenishes the spleen; *Ye Ju Hua* and *Gua Lou* remove toxins and disperse accumulations.

Finally, for the heat toxin accumulation syndrome, the main symptoms are rapid growth in the breast tumour with pain, sometimes accompanied by redness and swelling and even ulcerations with pus and a foul odour. *Qi* and blood are damaged with serious loss of healthy *qi*, manifesting as pallor and anaemia, weight loss, fatigue, feverishness and irritability, constipation, dry eyes and mouth, yellow-white or yellowish and greasy tongue fur, and a taut and slippery or taut and rapid pulse. The TCM therapeutic approach is to resolve toxins, improve blood circulation, and strengthen vital (healthy) *qi*. An appropriate prescription comprises *Mao Zhua Cao* 30 g, *Shan Ci Gu* 15 g, *Cao He Che* 15 g,

Liu Ji Nu 10 g, *Feng Fang* 10 g, *Pu Gong Ying* 30 g, *Quan Gua Lou* 30 g, *Sheng Di Huang* 15 g, *Xuan Shen* 12 g, *Dang Gui* 10 g, *Fu Rong Ye* 20 g and *Sheng Huang Qi* 30 g.

In advanced stages of cancer, deficiency of healthy *qi* co-exists with exuberance of pathogens. Thus, the treatment should reinforce vital (healthy) *qi* and dissipate pathogenic factors. We can use herbs that clear heat, relieve toxins, activate blood and dissipate stagnation. Meanwhile, we should reinforce vital *qi* especially when the tumour is ulcerated. We can tonify *qi* and nourish blood using such herbs as *Sheng Huang Qi, Sheng Di Huang* and *Dang Gui*, and prescriptions like *Gui Pi Tang, Xiang Bei Yang Rong Tang* and *Shi Quan Da Bu Tang*. The main therapeutic effect is that of tonifying *qi* and nourishing blood, with removing toxins and dissipating nodes playing a supplementary role.

Overall, the herbs commonly used to treat various syndromes associated with breast cancer are *Bai Ying, Pu Gong Ying, Long Kui, Tu Fu Ling, Ban Zhi Lian, She Mei, Xian Ren Zhang, Feng Fang, Ban Mao, Shan Dou Gen, Shan Ci Gu, Zhu Yang Yang, Tian Kui Zi, Lian Qiao, Zao Xiu, Fu Rong Hua, Bai Hua She She Cao, Zi Cao, Xia Ku Cao, Qing Pi, Gou Ju Li, Ze Lan, Liu Xing Zi, Zao Jiao Ci, Chuan Shan Jia, Xie Ke, Tian Men Dong, Xue Li Guo, Tian Hua Fen, Chuan Lian Zi, Ai Ye, Lou Lü, Tu Bei Mu, Ye Pu Tao Gen, Sheng Nan Xing, Sheng Ban Xia, Jiang Can, Sha Yuan Zi, Lao Ling Ke* and *Chou Chun Pi Gen*.

Fu Xiao Mai may be added when spontaneous sweating occurs; *Luo Shi Teng, Sang Zhi* and *Lu Lu Tong* when swelling appears in the arms; *Da Huang* and *Bai Zi Ren* for patients with constipation; *Ye Jiao Teng* and *Chao Zao Ren* for patients with poor sleep; *Chai Hu, Chi Shao, Yin Chen* and *Jiang Huang* if there are liver function disorders; and *Cao Jue Ming, Yin Chen* and *Ze Xie* for patients with fatty liver and obesity due to long-term use of tamoxifen.

Case 1

Female, 75 years old, ethnic han, married.

First visit: 6 June 1966
History of present illness: Tumour in the right breast, measuring 2.5 cm; histological examination proved it to be breast cancer. The patient had other chronic diseases such as hypertension, cardiac disease, hip joint problem and poor vision. She was not suitable for surgery, chemotherapy or radiotherapy. She was given tamoxifen 10 mg, twice a day.
Symptoms: Frequent and painful urination; red tongue tip; deep, thready and weak pulse.
Syndrome differentiation: Liver depression and *qi* stagnation, accumulation of phlegm and toxins.
TCM principle for treatment: Soothing the liver *qi*, strengthening the spleen, resolving phlegm and toxins.
Prescription: *Cu Chai Hu* 10 g, *Shan Ci Gu* 15 g, *Sheng Mu Li* 30 g, *Xia Ku Cao* 15 g, *Cao He Che* 15 g, *Wang Bu Liu Xing* 10 g, *Chi Shao* 10 g, *Ji Xue Teng* 30 g, *Du Zhong* 10 g, *Bai Hua She She Cao* 30 g, *Shan Yao* 30 g, *Sheng Huang Qi* 30 g, *Wu Yao* 10 g, *Qu Mai* 15 g, *Qian Hu* 10 g and *Pu Gong Ying* 15 g.

Visit three months later: Pain in the right breast was reduced; urination and appetite were improved; pale red tongue with thin white fur; deep, thready and wiry pulse.
The prescription was modified to *Xiang Fu* 10 g, *Yu Jin* 10 g, *Bei Sha Shen* 30 g, *Tian Hua Fen* 15 g, *Shan Ci Gu* 15 g, *Sheng Mu Li* 30 g, *Xia Ku Cao* 15 g, *Cao He Che* 15 g, *Chi Shao* 10 g, *Ji Xue Teng* 30 g, *Du Zhong* 10 g, *Tu Fu Ling* 15 g, *Sheng Huang Qi* 30 g, *Pu Gong Ying* 15 g, *Mai Dong* 15 g and *Wu Wei Zi* 10 g.

After three months of using the previous prescription, the patient's health improved. The patient occasionally felt pain in the chest, had good appetite and slept well, had normal bowel movements, and had a red tongue with yellow fur and a thready and slippery pulse.

Prescription: *Tai Zi Shen* 30 g, *Chuan Xiong* 10 g, *Tian Hua Fen* 15 g, *Chuan Lian Zi* 10 g, *Cao He Che* 15 g, *Huang Qin* 10 g, *Ji Xue Teng* 30 g, *Sha Yuan Zi* 10 g, *Sheng Huang Qi* 30 g, *Pu Gong Ying* 15 g, *Mai Dong* 15 g, *Wu Wei Zi* 10 g, *Bai Ying* 15 g and *Jiao San Xian* 10 g each.

After four months of using the previous prescription, the patient underwent a comprehensive check-up. The following was observed: thinning of the cortex for both kidneys, fatty liver, multiple cysts in the liver, a red tongue with thin yellow fur, and a deep and thready pulse. The patient felt no pain in the breast. The prescription was modified to *Shan Ci Gu* 15 g, *Sheng Mu Li* 30 g, *Xia Ku Cao* 15 g, *Tian Hua Fen* 15 g, *Cao He Che* 15 g, *Pao Shan Jia* 10 g, *Chi Shao* 10 g, *Ji Xue Teng* 30 g, *Du Zhong* 10 g, *Bai Hua She She Cao* 30 g, *Nü Zhen Zi* 15 g, *Sheng Huang Qi* 30 g, *Gou Qi Zi* 10 g, *Bai Ying* 20 g, *Long Kui* 15 g and *Pu Gong Ying* 15 g.

After seven months of using the previous prescription, no tumour in the right breast was found. After another eight months' treatment, a tumour in the right breast was detected; this was confirmed by examinations conducted in several other hospitals. TCM treatment continued; after two years on the prescription, no recurrence occurred.

Comments

This is a case of an elderly woman with a clear diagnosis of right breast cancer in the post-menopausal period. Given the condition of the patient, neither surgery, radiotherapy nor chemotherapy was used. Western treatment applied tamoxifen, whilst TCM treatment used soothing the liver, regulating *qi*, clearing heat and toxins, softening of accumulations and tonifying *qi* based on syndrome differentiation. The matching of the herbs to the syndromes helped to achieve satisfactory results, with no pain or symptoms of a breast tumour four years after a tumour had been diagnosed.

Case 2

Female, 63 years old, ethnic han, married, retired.

First visit: 17 June 2004
Main complaint: Three years after modified radical mastectomy in 2001, there were papillary adenocarcinoma, many vascular cancerous embolisms and 6/16 lymphatic node metastasis. Immunohistochemical analysis showed ER-, PR-, HER-2 +++.
Treatment history: The patient received modified radical mastectomy in June 2001. Radiotherapy was applied for three weeks after operation for a total of 25 times, then TAT+EPI chemotherapy for three weeks, without using tamoxifen. Recently, left-sided superclavicle lymph node metastasis was found, and local radiotherapy was applied 30 times.
Present symptoms: Distension and pain in the stomach; bitterness in the mouth; dryness in the throat; poor appetite; belching; occasional irritability; red tongue with yellow fur; and thin and taut pulse.
Western medical diagnosis: Lymph node metastasis; bone metastasis after breast cancer operation; fatty liver.

TCM syndrome differentiation: Disharmony of the liver and stomach, blood stasis and accumulation of toxins.

Principle for treatment: Soothing the liver and regulating the stomach, nourishing *yin* and detoxification.

Prescription: Xuan Fu Hua 10 g, Dai Zhe Shi 15 g, Zhi Ke 10 g, Hou Po 10 g, Chai Hu 10 g, Chi Shao 10 g, Tian Hua Fen 15 g, Ju Hua 10 g, Sha Shen 30 g, Mai Dong 15 g, Bai Zhu 10 g, Fu Ling 10 g, Ban Zhi Lian 15 g, Bai Hua She She Cao 30 g, Long Kui 15 g, Bai Ying 30 g, She Mei 15 g and Chao Zao Ren 20 g.

Next visit: 30 June 2004

Symptoms generally improved; appetite continued to be poor; spontaneous sweating; dark tongue with signs of blood stasis and thin, yellowish fur; thready and wiry pulse.

The prescription was modified: *Tian Hua Fen, Mai Dong* and *Ju Hua* were substituted with *Sheng Huang Qi* 30 g, *Fang Feng* 10 g and *Fu Xiao Mai* 30 g.

Next visit: 16 September 2004

Symptoms: Loose stools; poor sleep; belching; better appetite; darkish tongue with signs of blood stasis and whitish and yellow greasy fur; thin, slippery and rapid pulse.

Prescription: Xuan Fu Hua 10 g, Dai Zhu Shi 15 g, Chai Hu 10 g, Ze Xie 15 g, Yu Jin 10 g, Chuan Lian Zi 10 g, Chi Shao 10 g, Yin Chen 15 g, Cao Jue Ming 15 g, Huo Xiang 10 g, Zhi Zi 10 g, Zhi Ke 10 g, Bai Ying 30 g, Long Kui 15 g, She Mei 15 g, Bai Zhu 10 g, Fu Ling 10 g, Sheng Huang Qi 15 g, Jiao San Xian 10 g each and Sha Ren 10 g.

Next visit: 8 December 2004

Symptoms: Stomach discomfort and belching reduced, stools normal, distension and pain in the hepatic region, poor sleep quality.

Prescription: *Yuan Hu* 15 g and *Sha Yuan Zi* 10 g were added to the previous prescription.

During two further visits in February 2005, metastasis was found in the lymph nodes. The TCM prescription was modified to deal with this, and further adjustments were made in May and September 2005.

Next visit: 9 October 2005
There was no obvious change in the lymph nodes above the left collarbone.
Symptoms: General conditions were good; light red tongue with tooth indentations and thin white fur; deep and wiry pulse. Damp-heat and stagnation symptoms were alleviated.
Prescription: *Sha Shen* 30 g, *Sheng Huang Qi* 30 g, *Tai Zi Shen* 20 g, *Dang Shen* 10 g, *Ji Xue Teng* 30 g, *Nü Zhen Zi* 15 g, *Gou Qi Zi* 10 g, *Shan Yu Rou* 10 g, *Tian Hua Fen* 15 g, *Chi Bai Shao* 10 g each, *Zhe Bei Mu* 10 g, *Cao He Che* 15 g, *Bai Ying* 30 g, *Long Kui* 15 g, *She Mei* 15 g, *Dan Pi* 10 g, *Chao Zao Ren* 20 g, *Jiao San Xian* 10 g each, *Ji Nei Jin* 10 g and *Sha Ren* 10 g.

Next visit: 3 December 2005
Symptoms: Fatigue; dry throat; pale reddish tongue with thin white fur; deep, thready and weak pulse. Examination showed lymph nodes present in the sternal region, the largest being 1.1 cm × 0.75 cm.
Prescription: *Sheng Huang Qi* 30 g, *Dang Shen* 10 g, *Tai Zi Shen* 20 g, *Gou Qi Zi* 10 g, *Nü Zhen Zi* 15 g, *Mai Dong* 10 g, *Tian Hua Fen* 15 g, *Xia Ku Cao* 15 g, *Bai Zhu* 10 g, *Fu Ling* 10 g, *Bai Ying* 30 g, *Long Kui* 15 g, *She Mei* 15 g, *Bai Hua She She Cao* 30 g, *Cao He Che* 15 g, *Hai Zao* 15 g, *Jiao San Xian* 10 g each, *Ji Nei Jin* 10 g, *Sha Ren* 10 g, *Sha Yuan Zi* 10 g can add *Xi Huang Jiao Nan* (capsules).

Next visit: 18 March 2006

PET examination showed that nodes had formed (1.2 cm × 0.8 cm) in the suprasternal fossa, with possible metastasis; B-ultrasound showed lymph nodes in the suprasternal fossa (1.2 cm × 0.8 cm); radiotherapy and chemotherapy being considered by the Western doctor.

Prescription: Sha Shen 30 g, *Chuan Bei* 10 g, *Tian Hua Fen* 15 g, *Ju Ye* 10 g, *Sheng Huang Qi* 30 g, *Tai Zi Shen* 20 g, *Nü Zhen Zi* 15 g, *Gou Qi Zi* 10 g, *Ban Zhi Lian* 15 g, *Bai Hua She She Cao* 30 g, *Long Kui* 15 g, *Cao He Che* 15 g, *Bei Dou Gen* 6 g, *Sha Yuan Zi* 10 g, *Ji Xue Teng* 30 g, *Yuan Hu* 15 g, *Chao Zao Ren* 20 g, *Jiao San Xian* 10 g each, *Ji Nei Jin* 10 g and *Sha Ren* 10 g.

Next visit: 26 April 2006

Chemotherapy was started using CDDP, Navelbine and Herceptin. TCM treatment continued concurrently with chemotherapy.

Prescription: Sheng Huang Qi 30 g, *Tai Zi Shen* 20 g, *Dang Shen* 10 g, *Ji Xue Teng* 30 g, *Nü Zhen Zi* 15 g, *Gou Qi Zi* 10 g, *Shan Yu Rou* 10 g, *Zi He Che* 10 g, *Ci Wu Jia* 15 g, *Sha Ren* 10 g and *Da Zao* 6 g.

Next visit: 14 June 2006

Right supraclavicular lymph node metastasis, about 0.5 cm × 0.13 cm.

Symptoms: Abdominal distension, nausea and vomiting, loss of taste, dry stools, normal urination.

Prescription: Ji Xue Teng 30 g, *Zhe Bei Mu* 10 g, *Shan Yu Rou* 10 g, *Zi He Che* 10 g, *Ju Pi* 10 g, *Zhu Ru* 10 g, *Ban Xia* 10 g, *Ci Wu Jia* 15 g, *Chao Zao Ren* 20 g, *Sha Shen* 20 g, *Sha Yuan Zi* 10 g, *Dan Shen* 15 g, *Sheng Huang Qi* 30 g, *Tai Zi Shen* 30 g, *Dang Shen* 15 g, *Nü Zhen Zi* 15 g, *Gou Qi Zi* 10 g, *Tu Si Zi* 10 g, *Jiao San*

Xian 10 g each, *Ji Nei Jin* 10 g, *Sha Ren* 10 g, *Zhi Ke* 10 g and *Hou Po Hua* 10 g.

Comments

Although the tumour was resected, there was extensive lymph node metastasis (16/16). Immunohistochemical analysis showed strong positive c-*erb*B2 (+++). This case of breast cancer was vulnerable to metastasis which first showed up some three years after surgery. This could suggest that combining TCM treatment with radiotherapy and chemotherapy played a role in controlling metastasis.

Differentiation of syndromes indicated the use of different herbs and formulas to treat the TCM condition. Differentiation of diseases indicated treatment of the breast cancer according to specific characters of this disease by the Western medical approach. It was possible to improve the overall therapeutic results by combining differentiation of syndromes with differentiation of diseases.

Chemotherapy using Herceptin can have adverse effects such as fatigue, general pain, cough, digestive problems, rash, depression, insomnia, cough or asthma. TCM syndrome differentiation was used to reinforce vital *qi* to alleviate these side effects. This had the benefits of regulating *qi* and blood, balancing the five organs, tonifying and reinforcing vital *qi*, and dispersing toxins and pathogens. The patient's immune system was strengthened and quality of life improved, with a delay in the progression of metastasis.

In the course of dealing with this case, we made the useful discovery that the following prescription can be applied to treat fatty liver: *Yin Chen, Cao Jue Ming* and *Ze Xie.* The three herbs proved to be effective in reducing liver lipid levels.

5.3. Liver Cancer

Liver cancer consists of primary liver cancer and secondary liver cancer, also known as metastatic liver cancer. The latter occurs as a result of the spread of primary cancer from another location. Henceforth we use the term "liver cancer" to refer to primary hepatic cancer. This is one of the most common malignant tumours in China and other countries. Owing to their slow and insidious onset, most cases are not diagnosed until the middle or late stages when prognosis tends to be poorer.

In China, the mortality rate for liver cancer in urban areas ranks third, after lung cancer and gastric cancer, whilst in rural districts it is the second highest, after gastric cancer. Over 110,000 people die of the disease annually in China, accounting for over 40% of the total deaths worldwide from the disease. The incidence of the disease is particularly high in the north-east coastal provinces.

In classical Chinese medical literature, symptoms such as pain in the right trunk region near the liver, lumps, jaundice and bleeding typical of liver cancer are extensively recorded. From the TCM point of view, the primary pathogenic factors that contribute to liver cancer are the attack of exogenous cold, dampness and heat dampness combined with internal deficiencies of the spleen and stomach caused by improper diet; or depressed emotions cause stagnation of liver *qi* and and blood stasis, resulting in accumulation into a tumour; or spleen *yang* is suppressed by dampness, transforming into heat and resulting in jaundice. In sum, the pathogenesis of liver cancer comprises internal deficiencies of *qi* and blood, spleen deficiency with dampness, *qi* stagnation and blood stasis as well as attacks of external climatic pathogens and toxins invading the body, whose deficiencies cause it to succumb to the invasion and develop tumours as a result.

Epidemiological studies suggest that in regions with a high incidence of liver cancer, viruses and chemical carcinogens are additional external predisposing factors for the disease. Studies show that there is a close link between hepatic cancer and incidence of acute viral hepatitis; acute viral hepatitis can lead to chronic liver conditions and bring about liver cirrhosis which later transforms into cancer.

Among carcinogens, aflatoxin has been found to have high potency for inducing liver cancer. It can be found in peanuts, corn and other grains that have developed mildew. In addition, *Aspergillus* toxins, islandicin and luteoskyrin have been found to induce liver cancer in laboratory animals. Nitrosamines in certain foods are also thought to be carcinogenic.

Generally, the presence of external factors is a condition for the development of liver cancers, but the host body has to have inherent weaknesses and imbalances as outlined earlier for these external factors to take effect and induce cancerous tumours to form. Hence, a healthy immune system and the prevention of hepatitis and liver cirrhosis form the basic approach to defending against external influences and carcinogenic factors that bring about the disease.

5.3.1. TCM treatment by differentiating syndromes

The main syndromes accompanying patients with liver cancer are briefly described here:

1. Depression of liver *qi*.
2. *Qi* stagnation and blood stasis.
3. Coagulation of warm dampness.
4. Damage of liver *yin*.

The following two cases illustrate the fact that several of these syndromes can often be present at the same time, making the treatment of such complex combinations of syndromes more challenging for the TCM physician.

Case 1

Male, 38 years old, ethnic han.

First visit: 5 June 1987

Western medical diagnosis: Two months after resection for hepatocarcinoma, the patient had pain in the liver region. Primary liver cancer, cirrhosis.

History of present illness: The patient developed hepatitis B in 1974 and was diagnosed with cirrhosis in 1985. In October 1986, a space-occupying lesion measuring 1.3 cm × 1.6 cm was found by B-type ultrasonography in his right liver lobe. Exploratory laparotomy was performed in January 1987 but it was not possible to make a full examination of the lesion owing to nodular cirrhosis. Three months after the operation, the AFP reached 2300 ng/ml. The patient accepted surgery by resection of the right liver lobe. Pathological examination showed cirrhosis and primary liver cancer. After the surgery, the AFP of the patient decreased to 540 ng/ml.

TCM symptoms: Bright pale complexion, lassitude, poor appetite, sticky sensation in the mouth, slight nausea, hepatalgia, numbness in the tongue, distension of the eyeball. Dark red tongue, yellowish-white greasy fur; taut, thready and slippery pulse.

TCM syndrome differentiation: Retained warm toxins, stagnation of liver and gall bladder.

Treatment principle: Soothing the liver and promoting bile flow; resolving dampness and toxins.

Prescription: *Hu Zhang* 30 g, *Yu Jin* 10 g, *Tai Zi Shen* 30 g, *Ju Pi* 10 g, *Zhu Ru* 10 g, *Bai Zhu* 10 g, *Yun Ling* 10 g, *Tu Fu Ling* 20 g, *Pu Gong Ying* 20 g, *Shou Wu Teng* 30 g, *Chao Zao Ren* 15 g, *Jiao San Xian* 10 g each, *Ban Zhi Lian* 30 g, *Long Kui* 20 g, *Bai Hua She She Cao* 20 g, *Yu Zhi Zi* 15 g, *Zhi Qiao* 10 g and *Hou Po* 10 g. Fourteen doses were prescribed.

Next visit: 29 June 1987
The patient increased his food intake. Abdominal distension and hepatalgia were reduced. However, a re-examination using B-type ultrasonography found a space-occupying lesion of around 1.6 cm × 1.2 cm in the left liver lobe. The tongue and pulse were unchanged since the last examination. The prescription was modified to eliminate *Ju Pi*, *Zhu Ru*, *Pu Gong Ying*, *Chao Zao Ren* and *Jiao San Xian*. Another 14 doses were prescribed.

Next visit: 13 July 1987
Symptoms: Moderate food intake, tinnitus, occasional dull pain in the hepatic region, loose stools. Dark red enlarged tongue with tooth indentations. AFP: 25 ng/ml.

Syndrome pattern: Liver depression and spleen deficiency, retained heat toxins.

Treatment method: Soothing the liver and fortifying the spleen, clearing away heat and removing toxic substances.

Prescription: *Dang Shen* 14 g, *Bai Zhu* 10 g, *Fu Ling* 10 g, *Chen Pi* 10 g, *Hou Pou* 10 g, *Hang Shao* 10 g, *Mu Xiang* 10 g, *Yu Jin* 10 g, *Hu Zhang* 30 g, *Tu Fu Ling* 20 g, *Chao Zhi Zi* 15 g, *Ban Zhi Lian* 30 g, *Bai Hua She She Cao* 30 g, *Chao Zao Ren* 20 g, *Shou Wu Teng* 20 g and *Jiao San Xian* 10 g each.

The patient took this prescription for half a month and his AFP dropped below 25 ng/ml, which was within the normal range. Food intake increased but hepatalgia persisted and sleep was poor. The prescription was maintained until 14 September 1987. Re-examination indicated that the lesion in the left liver had disappeared and the AFP had dropped to 25 ng/ml.

From October 1987 to April 1988, the patient took a decoction based on the earlier prescription with slight modifications. Apart from occasional hepatalgia, the patient felt normal in terms of food intake, sleep, urine and stools. He was deemed to be in a stable state.

Date of visit: 6 May 1988
Patient complained of tinnitus, dizzy vision, poor food intake, dry mouth, poor sleep and dry stools. General signs: dark red dry tongue with thin whitish fur; taut and thready pulse.
Syndrome pattern: Liver and kidney deficiency.
Therapeutic method: Nourishing the kidney and fortifying the liver.
Prescription: *Sheng Shu Di* 10 g each, *Shan Yao* 10 g, *Shan Yu Rou* 15 g, *Sha Ren* 10 g, *Mu Xiang* 10 g, *Yuan Zhi* 10 g, *Fu Ling* 10 g, *Dan Pi* 10 g, *Ze Xie* 10 g, *Tian Hua Fen* 15 g, *Tu Fu Ling* 20 g, *Hu Zhang* 20 g, *Yuan Hu* 10 g, *Jiao San Xian* 10 g each, *Ban Zhi Lian* 30 g, *Bai Hua She She Cao* 30 g, *Sheng Huang Qi* 20 g and *Nü Zhen Zi* 12 g.

After the patient was on this prescription for more than one month, all symptoms except occasional hepatalgia were relieved. From then on, the patient visited every two months. Some modifications to the prescription were made as appropriate to the symptoms each time. A follow-up visit in November 1990 indicated that he was in stable condition in general and lived a normal daily life. Re-examination showed that his AFP was lower than 25 ng/ml (negative). B-sonography found no space-occupying lesion in the left liver lobe.

Comments

TCM uses syndrome differentiation and treatment as the basic approach. Though the primary cancer was removed by surgery, the syndrome pattern of the patient was in a dynamic state. After the resection, the patient first manifested retained warm toxin syndrome. When the toxins were cleared, the patient presented liver depression and spleen deficiency syndrome which later progressed to liver and kidney deficiency. The patient's state transformed from an excess syndrome to a deficiency syndrome, although it should be noted that the deficiency existed even from the very beginning but was concealed by the damp-heat and liver depression. When the damp-heat and liver depression syndromes had been alleviated, the deficiency syndrome manifested itself more clearly.

This case received effective treatment in part because of the combination of correct syndrome differentiation and appropriate medication.

A guiding principle in the treatment process for such cases is to address the acute syndrome first and the milder, more deeply rooted syndrome over the longer term. This principle is especially relevant in cancer cases, which commonly have deficiency-excess complex syndromes. The patient initially had symptoms like a bright pale complexion, lassitude, poor appetite and a thready pulse, indicating spleen qi deficiency syndrome; on the other hand, he also had a sticky sensation in the mouth, slight nausea, hepatalgia, numbness in the tongue, distension of the eyeballs and yellowish-white greasy fur, suggesting the presence of liver and gallbladder damp-heat syndrome. Careful analysis suggested that damp-heat in the liver and gallbladder was the main condition requiring primary attention for treatment. As a result, elimination of damp-heat in the liver and gallbladder was set as the major treatment method and fortifying the spleen was selected as the complementary one. After the damp-heat pathogen was cleared and liver depression alleviated, the patient started to exhibit pronounced symptoms associated with liver *yin* deficiency syndrome. Hence, a variation of the classic *yin* deficiency decoction *Liu Wei Di Huang Wan* was prescribed.

Combining the holistic syndrome differentiation of TCM and the diagnostic techniques of modern medicine at the microscopic level was the integrated approach taken in managing this case. In addition to observing external symptoms and syndromes and the use of B-sonography, indices of liver function, AFP and other microscopic indicators were also closely studied. This combined system enabled TCM to achieve a higher level of effectiveness in therapy.

Case 2

Male, 31 years old, ethnic han.

First visit: 13 July 1989
Main complaint: Abdominal distension for four months.
History of present illness: The patient started to experience a pricking pain in the right hypochondrium in January 1989. The pain lasted for several minutes and was recurrent. B-sonography and CT scan at Beijing Chaoyang Hospital suggested that there were space-occupying lesions in the liver.

Exploratory laparotomy found bloody ascites in the abdominal cavity, an enlarged liver and gallbladder, and a mass in the right liver lobe (15 cm × 15 cm). Owing to the fact that the tumour had extensively invaded the surrounding liver tissue, resection could not be done. A pathologic specimen was taken and chemotherapy with 5-FU (500 mg) was administered. After the operation, the patient was not given further chemotherapy or radiotherapy. The pathology report indicated hepatoma.

B-sonography: The liver had an irregular surface and its internal parts generated an unbalanced echo. The right liver lobe deviated to the left. Several solid masses were detected in the liver, the largest being 7.8 cm × 6.5 cm.

Liver function tests: Jaundice index: 30 units.

Van den Bergh test: Direct biphasic reaction.

GPT: 214 units.

Western medical diagnosis: Primary liver cancer, cirrhosis, ascites.

TCM examination: Pale darkish tongue with yellowish fur; taut, slippery pulse; jaundiced face. The diagnosis was tympanites (distension of the abdomen).

Syndrome pattern: Liver depression and spleen deficiency, dampness in the "middle energizer" (*zhongjiao*) of the trunk.

Therapeutic method: Soothing the liver and fortifying the spleen; resolving dampness and jaundice.

Prescription: Yin Chen 15 g, Jin Qian Cao 30 g, Yu Jin 10 g, Jiang Huang 10 g, Sheng Huang Qi 30 g, Bai Zhu 10 g, Fu Ling 10 g, Mu Xiang 10 g, Zhu Ling 15 g, Ze Xie 12 g, Chuan Pu 10 g, Zhi Qiao 10 g, Ban Bian Lian 30 g, Da Fu Pi 10 g, Chou Hu Lu 20 g, Che Qian Cao 30 g, Sha Ren 10 g, Zhi Zi 10 g, Bai Xian Pi 15 g, Chang Pu 15 g and Ji Nei Jin 10 g.

Second visit: 20 July 1987

Appetite improved, and stool formation was regular. Symptoms like jaundice, oedema and hydroperitonia were as before. Pale reddish enlarged tongue with thin whitish fur; taut, thready and slightly rapid pulse. Syndrome differentiation and therapeutic principles were unchanged.

Prescription: The earlier prescription was modified, with *Rou Gui* 2 g, *Chao Zhi Bai* 10 g each and *Yuan Hu* 20 g added.

The prescription adopted in the second visit continued in subsequent visits but the *Long She Yang Quan* decoction (*Long Kui* 30 g, *Bai Hua She She Cao* 30 g, *Bai Ying* 30 g) was added.

Date of visit: 26 October 1989 (27 months later)

The patient had taken more than 70 doses of TCM medication. His condition was much improved and he was in better spirits, with good food intake and without abdominal bloating. His stool formation was regular and urine was normal. His tongue was pale red and enlarged, and his pulse was thready, slippery and slightly rapid. Physical examination showed that the colour of the skin was normal; the sclera was slightly yellowish; the sublingual mucous membranes were normal; a slightly dark complexion; the abdomen was flat; ascites (+++) under the ribs on the liver side and the spleen side. The lower limbs were without oedema. B-sonography showed the liver had an irregular surface and generated an unbalanced echo. Several solid masses could be detected in the liver, the largest being 6 cm × 7 cm; some of them with dark fluid; small degree of ascites.

Comments

Late-stage cancerous ascites are quite difficult to deal with clinically. The patient, suffering from advanced hepatoma, developed severe jaundice on top of ascites, making it extremely difficult to treat. The courses of TCM medication prescribed in this case demonstrated the three key principles of managing such advanced cancers:

1. Differentiate the syndrome pattern of the patient at each stage and select herbs accordingly. The patient's initial symptoms of a dark complexion, jaundice of a yellowish-green hue, loss of appetite, ill-formed stools, abdominal bloating, dark yellow and scanty urine, and a pale and enlarged tongue were consistent with liver depression, spleen deficiency and accumulation of dampness in middle-energizer syndromes. Soothing the liver and fortifying the spleen to resolve dampness and jaundice were the main therapeutic objectives at this stage. At the second visit, the patient experienced improved food intake, indicating recovery of spleen *qi* and alleviation of liver depression. Symptoms of a dark complexion, an enlarged tongue and poorly formed stools suggested *yang-qi* deficiency syndrome, and dark yellow and scanty urine pertained to the syndrome of damp-heat in the lower energizer. The earlier prescription was supplemented with *Rou Gui* 2 g and *Chao Zhi Bai* 10 g each. *Rou Gui* warms kidney *yang* and enriches spleen *yang*, and thus fortifies the dampness transportation and transformation function of the spleen and the water-governing function of the kidney.

2. Holistic approach to symptoms. As in the previous case, the patient manifested a deficiency-excess complex syndrome. The more acute syndrome was dealt with first. On one hand, *yin* and *yang* were in disharmony, and there was deficiency in *qi* and blood; on the other hand, there were

excess symptoms of abdominal masses, ascites and pain. During the first visit, inducing diuresis to alleviate bloating alone would have been too drastic and risked damaging healthy *qi*; merely reinforcing healthy *qi* would not have been sufficient to remove the dampness. Thus, herbs fortifying the spleen such as *Fu Ling*, *Bai Zhu* and *Ji Nei Jin* were supplemented with *Da Fu Pi*, *Che Qian Cao*, *Chou Hu Lu*, *Yin Chen* and *Jin Qian Cao* to resolve dampness and eliminate jaundice.

3. Clinical experience is essential for the correct management of complex syndromes seen in cancer patients. In the first stage of treatment of this patient, it was decided based on clinical experience that the deficiency syndrome would receive priority attention, whilst at the same time taking steps to deal with pathogenic factors. The decoction *Long She Yang Quan* which combats cancerous pathogens was used next to restore healthy *qi*, drawing on the principle that the body would on its own restore healthy *qi* after pathogenic factors were removed.

5.4. Colorectal Cancer

Colorectal cancer includes colon cancer and rectal cancer, and is one of the most common forms of cancer. Most cases occur above the age of 45; the disease affects both men and women, although its incidence is higher among males.

TCM differentiates a number of syndromes associated with colorectal cancer, occurring singly or in combination:

1. Deficiency of the spleen with warm dampness. The patient has a poor appetite, bloated abdomen, yellow pallor, shortness of breath and lassitude, pain in the abdomen alleviated

by pressure, diarrhoea, blood in the stools, yellow greasy fur, and a slippery and rapid or deep and thready pulse. The therapeutic approach is to fortify the spleen and regulate *qi*, dissipate heat and resolve dampness.

2. Warm dampness with accumulation of toxins. The patient's abdomen is bloated and there is pain which is alleviated by pressure; there may be a lumpy mass in the lower abdomen. Bloating is reduced with release of wind. Other symptoms include diarrhoea or loose stools, a darkish red tongue with ecchymosis (purple spot) and thin yellow fur, and a taut and rapid pulse. The therapeutic principle is to use herbs to dissipate heat and resolve toxins; regulate *qi* and alleviate *qi* stagnation; resolve stasis and shrink masses.

3. Spleen-kidney cold dampness. The patient typically has frequent diarrhoea for a long period of time, looks emaciated and pale in the face, suffers from lassitude and prefers to rest; he has pain in the abdomen which feels better when heat is applied. He is afraid of cold, has white fur on his tongue, and his pulse is deep, thready and weak. He would be diagnosed as having deficiency of spleen and kidney *yang* and cold dampness that accumulates toxins. Treatment consists of warming the kidney, fortifying the spleen and dissipating cold and dampness.

The best treatment results are achieved by a combination of Western methods with TCM medications. Depending on the stage of the cancer, surgery or surgery followed by chemotherapy/radiotherapy may be prescribed; herbal medications can be used concurrently or after surgery and chemotherapy/radiotherapy.

The following two cases illustrate some of the combination methods used.

Case 1

Female, 60 years old, ethnic han.

First visit: 25 June 1987

Chief complaint: Five months after colostomy due to sigmoid colon cancer, the patient had a fever for more than ten days.

History of current illness: In November 1986, the patient visited a hospital in Beijing for persistent pain in the abdomen for half a month in addition to frequent discharge of clear and loose stools with blood and pus for one week. A lump in the abdomen was detected on physical examination. Exploratory laparotomy was carried out on 20 January 1987, during which a tumour on the posterior abdominal wall was found at the junction of the sigmoid colon and rectum. Excision could not be done, so colostomy was performed and an abdominal pouch installed to replace anal discharge. Biopsy showed that the lump was sigmoid colon adenocarcinoma. Chemotherapy with 5-fluorouracil was administered ten times but halted in March 1987 because of severe side effects. In May the same year, the patient began having abdominal pain, distension and excessive sweating which were not effectively controlled by the Chinese medication received. On 14 June the patient had a sudden onset of fever reaching 39.6°. Antibiotics did not resolve the fever. At this point, the patient came to me for consultation.

Present symptoms: Low fever of 37.3°, abdominal pain, perspiration and fear of cold. Occasional cough with little phlegm; normal appetite and urination; pale yellowish dull complexion and sickly looking; dark tongue with purple spots and tooth indentations; tongue with white fur and yellowish greasy coating at the root; thready and slippery pulse. White blood count: 13.7×10^9/L.

TCM syndrome differentiation: *Qi* and blood deficiency with stagnation of warm dampness.

Therapeutic method: Clearing heat, removing dampness, resolving toxins and stasis.

Prescription: Modified *San Ren* Decoction. *Sheng Yi Mi* 15 g, *Xing Ren* 10 g, *Bai Kou Ren* 10 g, *Ban Xia* 12 g, *Hou Po* 10 g, *Huo Xiang* 10 g, *Pu Gong Ying* 30 g, *Tu Fu Ling* 20 g, *Huang Bai* 10 g, *Yuan Hu* 10 g, *Jiao San Xian* (*Jiao Mai Ya, Jiao Shen Qu, Jiao Shan Zha*) 10 g each, *Yin Hua* 20 g, *Chi Shao* 10 g, *Dan Pi* 10 g, *Gan Cao* 6 g and *Bai Hua She She Cao* 30 g (total of seven doses).

Second visit: 2 July 1987
After the first course of medication, abdominal pain was alleviated, damp toxins were partially resolved and fever subsided. The patient still had dull abdominal pain, spontaneous sweating, lassitude, poor appetite, indigestion and heart palpitations, and was in low spirits. The tongue was red with purple spots, with a white and greasy coating; the pulse was thready and slippery. The therapeutic method was maintained, with a slight modification to the medication as follows: *Yin Hua* and *Pu Gong Ying* were replaced by anti-cancer herbs *Cao He Che* 30 g and *Long Kui* 30 g; *Sheng Huang Qi* 20 g and *Sha Shen* 30 g were added to strengthen *qi* (14 doses were prescribed, one per day).

Third visit: 16 July 1987
Abdominal distension and pain were greatly reduced, but the patient still experienced dizziness and spontaneous sweating. Appetite and indigestion were improved while stools and urine were normal. The tongue was dark red with purple spots, a white coating and a yellowish-white greasy root; the pulse was thready, slippery and weak.

Prescription: The previous prescription was modified by adding *Ban Zhi Lian* 30 g and *Bai Tou Weng* 20 g (20 more doses).

Date of further consultation: 10 August 1987
The patient was in better physical condition and in higher spirits, according to her own assessment. She still had a poor appetite; stools and urine were normal; the tongue still had purple spots, a thin white coating and a slightly yellow root; the pulse was deep and thready.
Therapeutic method: Strengthening the spleen and removing dampness, resolving toxins.
Prescription: *Sha Shen* 30 g, *Tai Zi Shen* 30 g, *Sheng Huang Qi* 20 g, *Yun Ling* 10 g, *Tu Fu Ling* 20 g, *Sheng Yi Ren* 15 g, *Ban Xia* 10 g, *Jiao San Xian* 10 g each, *Chuan Lian Zi* 10 g, *Hou Po* 10 g, *Cao He Che* 15 g, *Long Kui* 30 g, *Bai Ying* 30 g, *She Mei* 20 g, *Ban Zhi Lian* 30 g and *Gan Cao* 6 g.

From August 1987 to March 1990, the patient mainly took the aforementioned decoction with slight modifications according to the symptoms exhibited. For example, when there were loose and clear stools, *Dou* and *Bu Gu Zhi* were added; when there were clear signs of heat and dampness, *Bai Tou Weng*, *Qing Pi* and *Bai Hua She She Cao* were added.

Date of further consultation: 19 March 1990
The ALT level was 51. The patient had a good appetite and no signs of weak breathing or excessive sweating. She continued to suffer occasionally from diarrhoea caused by inappropriate diet. She moved her bowels four to five times a day and was sensitive to cold. The tongue was a healthier light red with a thin white coating.

Treatment principle: Strengthening the spleen and fortifying *qi*; smoothening the liver and regulating the stomach; resolving the dampness and toxins.

Prescription: *Yin Chen* 15 g, *Huang Qin* 10 g, *Chai Hu* 10 g, *Yu Jin* 10 g, *Huang Lian* 10 g, *Sheng Yi Ren* 15 g, *Bai Kou Ren* 10 g, *Shan Yao* 10 g, *Sheng Huang Qi* 30 g, *Dang Shen* 15 g, *Cao He Che* 15 g, *Bai Ying* 30 g, *Long Kui* 30 g, *Hang Shao* 15 g, *Tu Fu Ling* 20 g, *Sheng Gan Cao* 6 g and *Bai Hua She She Cao* 30 g.

After this course of medication, the patient was generally in satisfactory condition. She passed formed stools two to three times a day without abdominal pain; liver functions appeared normal; and there were no unusual discharges from the original location of the anus. She had a ruddy complexion, a slightly dark tongue with a thin white coating, and a thready and slippery pulse. *Yin Chen* was removed from the formula and *Cang Bai Zhu* 10 g, *Shan Yu Rou* 10 g and *Gou Qi Zi* 10 g were added to invigorate the spleen and kidney.

From then on, the patient visited the doctor once or twice a year for the next ten years or so. Each examination detected no sign of relapse or metastasis. The patient had taken the herbal decoction consistently for 13 years and stopped only in the year 2000. In 2001, she had a fall and fractured her leg, and recovered after treatment. When I asked about the patient in June 2006, I discovered that, at 79 years old, she was well though physically not very mobile; her other symptoms were stable.

Comments

The patient accepted one course of chemotherapy but stopped because she could not tolerate the side effects. From then on, she took TCM herbal decoctions to manage her illness for 13 years, living with her cancer and seeing an improvement in her Karnofsky Performance Status (KPS) from 60 to 90.

At each stage, the patient received therapy based on TCM syndrome differentiation, taking into account both principal and secondary syndromes with appropriate priority placed on the treatment of each. In the initial stages of treatment, accumulation of heat dampness and toxins were the primary syndromes addressed. After the pathogens causing these excess syndromes were gradually removed, the deficiency syndromes, especially spleen-kidney deficiency, became the main target of remedy. Thus, spleen-strengthening, *qi*-reinforcing and methods for invigorating the kidney and spleen were applied. In addition, herbs with heat-removing, toxin-dissolving and anti-cancer functions (such as *Ban Zhi Lian, Bai Hua She She Cao, Teng Li Gen, E Zhu, Tu Fu Ling* and *Bai Tou Weng*) were used to inhibit the progression of the cancer. The course of therapy combined disease differentiation with syndrome differentiation. It also strengthened healthy *qi* while building body resistance to combat the development of the tumour. *Qi* reinforcement and invigoration of the spleen and kidney were the major methods for building up healthy *qi* whilst for resisting tumour growth, we used the methods of expelling toxins by dissipating heat, regulating *qi* and clearing stagnation, removing dampness to regulate the stomach, resolving stasis, and removing mass accumulations.

After December 1987, the management of the patient's condition was focused on symptoms of lassitude, poor appetite and digestion, spontaneous sweating, disturbed sleep, loose stools, a thready, slippery and weak pulse, and a dark tongue with purple spots. These symptoms were associated with the syndrome pattern of *qi* deficiency and blood stasis. As a result, she was further treated by kidney-spleen invigoration and the elimination of stasis and toxins. The results were encouraging. The patient was in a stable condition and relaxed state of mind, enjoying better appetite and sleep, leading almost a normal life. She insisted on continuing with the decoction daily until 2000 when she reduced it to three doses each week for another five years to consolidate her recovery.

Case 2

Male, 52 years old, ethnic han, married.

First visit: 22 October 1999

Main complaint: Nausea and poor appetite two months after cancer surgery.

History of current illness: The patient accepted resection due to transverse colon cancer on 16 August 1999. Biopsy indicated that it was moderately differentiated adenocarcinoma without lymphatic metastasis. Two courses of chemotherapy were administered after surgery. (The patient suffered from diabetes mellitus and hyperlipidaemia several years ago.)

Present TCM symptoms: Nausea; poor appetite; normal stools; tongue dark red with purple spots, crack lines in the middle, and white and slightly thick fur; deep and taut pulse.

TCM syndrome differentiation: *Qi* deficiency with blood stasis. The patient was deficient in healthy *qi* and suffering from blood stasis caused by damage to *qi* and blood from surgery and further aggravated by chemotherapy.

Therapeutic principle: Tonifying *qi* and activating blood, resolving stasis and detoxifying.

While chemotherapy was in progress, the following prescription was used: *Sheng Huang Qi* 30 g, *Tai Zi Shen* 30 g, *Bai Zhu* 10 g, *Fu Ling* 10 g, *Sheng Yi Mi* 15 g, *E Zhu* 10 g, *Ji Xue Teng* 30 g, *Dan Shen* 15 g, *Jiao San Xian* 10 g each, *Ji Nei Jin* 10 g, *Sha Ren* 10 g, *Nü Zhen Zi* 15 g, *Gou Qi Zi* 10 g, *Shan Yu Rou* 10 g and *Cao He Che* 15 g.

Date of further consultation: 5 November 1999
After chemotherapy, white blood count was lower than normal. Symptoms: poor appetite and food intake; lassitude; dark red tongue with thin whitish fur; taut, slippery and rapid pulse.
Prescription: *Sheng Huang Qi* 30 g, *Tai Zi Shen* 30 g, *Bai Zhu* 10 g, *Fu Ling* 10 g, *E Zhu* 10 g, *Ji Xue Teng* 30 g, *Tian Hua Fen* 15 g, *Cao Jue Ming* 15 g, *Nü Zhen Zi* 15 g, *Gou Qi Zi* 10 g, *Shan Yu Rou* 10 g, *Xian Ling Pi* 10 g, *Jiao San Xian* 10 g each, *Ji Nei Jin* 10 g, *Sha Ren* 10 g and *Zhi Gan Cao* 6 g.

Date of further consultation: 11 August 2000
One year after surgery, the patient was generally in normal condition except for occasional abdominal pains. Appetite was satisfactory; urine and stools were normal; tongue was dark red with a thin whitish coating; pulse was deep, thready and taut. Blood test showed that WBC was 4200/mm^3.
Prescription: *Teng Li Gen* 15 g, *Bai Hua She She Cao* 30 g, *Bai Ying* 30 g, *Long Kui* 20 g, *Bai Zhu* 10 g, *Fu Ling* 10 g, *Tu Fu Ling* 15 g, *Dang Shen* 15 g, *Sheng Huang Qi* 30 g, *Gou Qi Zi* 10 g, *Nü Zhen Zi* 15 g, *Jiao San Xian* 10 g each, *Ji Nei Jin* 10 g and *Zhi Gan Cao* 6 g.

Date of further consultation: 31 October 2003
After the operation, the patient had decoctions based on modifications of the aforementioned formula consistently for

four years to manage his disease. Recent re-examination showed no abnormal signs. The patient was normal in terms of diet, sleep, urine and stools. Examination showed a dark tongue with thin whitish fur and a taut, deep pulse.

Prescription: Sheng Huang Qi 30 g, Tai Zi Shen 30 g, Ji Xue Teng 30 g, Dan Shen 15 g, E Zhu 10 g, Cao He Che 15 g, Nü Zhen Zi 15 g, Gou Qi Zi 10 g, Tu Fu Ling 15 g, Bai Hua She She Cao 30 g, Jiao San Xian 10 g each and Sha Ren 10 g.

Date of further consultation: 2 February 2005
Six years after his operation, the patient was in stable and satisfactory condition. The previous prescription was maintained without *E Zhu*, with three doses per week.

Comments

While the patient was under chemotherapy, the physician chose replenishing *qi* and nourishing blood, fortifying the spleen and tonifying the kidney as the main therapeutic approach to alleviate the adverse side effects of chemotherapy and to protect the blood-building function of the bone marrow and the digestive functions of the stomach and spleen. This in all likelihood helped the patient complete his chemotherapy treatment plan successfully. When the patient's haemogram (blood picture) was poor, *Zi He Che, Lu Jiao Jiao, Gui Ban Jiao* and other tonifying herbs were added. With the assistance of these decoctions, the patient went through the chemotherapy course without abnormal events.

After the chemotherapy the treatment principle was shifted to a combination of reinforcing healthy *qi* and eliminating pathogenic factors. On the one hand, fortifying the spleen and tonifying the kidney were selected to be the main method of reinforcing healthy *qi*, the kidney being the origin of innate healthy *qi* endowment while the spleen is the source of acquired healthy *qi* endowment. On the other hand, clearing heat, dissolving toxins and removing stasis was the major method for eliminating pathogenic factors. To manage the colon cancer, the physician chose to use *Teng Li Gen, Bai Hua She She Cao, Bai Ying, Long Kui, She Mei, Tu Fu Ling* and other herbs. The prescription of 11 August 2000 is the most commonly used one for post-operation patients under chemotherapy.

The patient enjoyed a stable condition after taking herbal decoctions over the long term. The prescription was later simplified with fewer herbs, although maintaining the principle of combining the reinforcement of healthy *qi* with eliminating pathogenic factors. The patient was in better health and re-examinations every half a year showed nothing significantly unusual. He continued to take a maintenance dose of decoction every two days.

5.5. Stomach Cancer

Although the term "stomach cancer" is not used in the Chinese medical classics, there are extensive references to this condition in various ancient texts. The *Huangdi neijing* (*Lingshu*) describes the condition of a bloated abdomen, abdominal pain near the heart, difficulty swallowing and food obstruction, while the Han dynasty medical master Zhang Zhongjing's *Jinkui yaolüe* uses the term "*fanwei*" to describe the symptoms of vomiting after morning and evening meals and difficulty digesting food.

In modern TCM theory, the basic origins of stomach cancer are attributed to inappropriate dietary habits, worry and anxiety, disorder in the spleen functions, stagnation of *qi* and accumulation of phlegm. The syndrome patterns associated with stomach cancer are as follows:

1. Disharmony between the liver and the stomach. The common symptoms for this syndrome are a bloated abdomen with occasional pain spreading to the ribs, bitterness in the mouth, a vexatious feeling in the chest, belching, reduced appetite and food intake or vomiting, thin yellowish or white fur on the tongue, and a taut, thready pulse. The therapeutic principle for this syndrome is to soothe the liver and regulate the stomach, suppress the reverse flow of food and reduce pain.
2. Cold deficiency of the stomach and spleen. The symptoms are dull gnawing pain in the stomach and abdomen which is partly relieved with pressure and heat, occasional vomiting of clear fluids, a pale and dull complexion, cold limbs, tiredness and lacking in spirit, loose stools, a pale and swollen tongue with tooth indentations, white moist fur on the tongue, and a deep and slow or deep and thready pulse. The therapeutic principle is to warm the stomach, fortify the spleen and regulate the stomach.
3. Stagnation caused by accumulated toxins with blood stasis and stomach heat. Typical symptoms are stabbing pain in the stomach, pain with a feeling of heat, increased pain after ingesting food, dry mouth and thirst, abdominal sensitivity to pressure, and a lump below the heart region. Occasionally there is vomiting of blood or blood in the stools, dry skin, a dark purplish tongue with spots, and a deep and taut or thready and astringent pulse. The therapeutic principle is to eliminate toxins and resolve stasis, clear heat and nourish *yin*.

4. *Qi* and blood debility. This syndrome tends to happen at a late stage of stomach cancer when the body is severely anaemic. Symptoms include a pale and swollen face, lassitude, palpitations and shortness of breath, dizziness and blurred vision, insomnia, spontaneous sweating, loss of appetite, body emaciation, a palpable lumpy mass in the upper abdomen, a pale and fat tongue with white fur, and a weak, thready pulse. The therapeutic principle is to tonify *qi* and nourish blood, fortify the spleen and invigorate the kidney.

We consider two cases of stomach cancer that exhibit some of these syndromes.

Case 1

Male, 77 years old, ethnic han.

First visit: 1 March 2002
Chief complaint: Difficulty swallowing, chest tightness and discomfort after meals. Carcinoma of the cardia (opening of the oesophagus into the stomach) diagnosed 40 days ago.
History of present illness: Patient had difficulty swallowing in January 2002 and was diagnosed with a tumour. The biopsy histological report indicated adenocarcinoma of the cardia, part of it suggesting signet-ring cell carcinoma. On 24 January 2002 abdominal exploration discovered that 3 cm of the oesophagus was hardened. Round nodes of different sizes were found on the left liver, ranging from 0.2 cm to 0.8 cm. The surgical procedure was terminated because of an excessive drop in blood pressure. The diagnosis was carcinoma of the lower part of the oesophagus with spread to the liver. Radiotherapy and chemotherapy were not administered

because of the advanced age of the patient. In March 2002 he came to the hospital with symptoms of difficulty swallowing and discomfort after meals; urine and bowel movements were normal.

Present TCM symptoms: Deep red tongue with yellow fur; pulse thready and taut.

TCM syndrome differentiation: Deficiency of the spleen and stomach, phlegm and blood stagnation.

Therapeutic principle: Reinforcing the spleen and invigorating *qi*, removing toxins to resist cancer.

Prescription: *Xiao Ye Jin Qian Cao* 20 g, *Jiang Huang* 12 g, *Bai Ying* 30 g, *Long Kui* 15 g, *Bai Hua She She Cao* 30 g, *Tu Fu Ling* 15 g, *Cao He Che* 15 g, *Bai Zhu* 10 g, *Fu Ling* 10 g, *Tai Zi Shen* 30 g, *Sheng Huang Qi* 30 g, *Gou Qi Zi* 12 g, *Ji Xue Teng* 30 g, *Jiao San Xian* 30 g each, *Ji Nei Jin* 10 g and *Sha Ren* 10 g (one dose per day).

Subsequent visit: 29 March 2002

The symptoms were reduced.

The prescription followed the same therapeutic principle with some modifications: *Bai Ying* 30 g, *Long Kui* 20 g, *She Mei* 15 g, *Cao He Che* 15 g, *Teng Li Gen* 20 g, *Sheng Huang Qi* 30 g, *Tai Zi Shen* 30 g, *Mai Dong* 15 g, *Wu Wei Zi* 10 g, *Jiang Huang* 12 g, *Tu Fu Ling* 15 g, *Bai Zhu* 10 g, *Gou Qi Zi* 10 g, *Jiao San Xian* 10 g each, *Ji Nei Jin* 10 g and *Sha Ren* 10 g.

Date of visit: 17 May 2002

The patient's situation was stable, with good appetite, no difficulty swallowing, normal urination and defecation, a deep red tongue with thin white fur, and a deep, thready pulse.

Prescription: *Bai Ying* 30 g, *Long Kui* 20 g, *She Mei* 15 g, *Teng Li Gen* 20 g, *Bai Zhu* 10 g, *Fu Ling* 10 g, *Jiang Huang* 12 g, *Sheng*

Huang Qi 30 g, *Tai Zi Shen* 30 g, *Gou Qi Zi* 10 g, *Ji Nei Jin* 10 g, *Sha Ren* 10 g, *Jiao San Xian* 10 g each, *Bai Hua She She Cao* 30 g, *Tu Fu Ling* 15 g and *Da Zao* 6 pieces.

Date of visit: 14 June 2002
The situation was stable with no special new symptoms.
Prescription: *Sha Shen* 30 g, *Tai Zi Shen* 30 g, *Sheng Huang Qi* 30 g, *Ji Xue Teng* 30 g, *Teng Li Gen* 20 g, *Bai Ying* 30 g, *Long Kui* 20 g, *She Mei* 15 g, *Bai Hua She She Cao* 30 g, *Jiao San Xian* 10 g each, *Ji Nei Jin* 10 g, *Sha Ren* 10 g and *Cao Zao Ren* 20 g.

Subsequent visit: 8 October 2002
Normal appetite, good sleep, normal urination and bowel movements, dark red tongue with thin white fur, deep and thready pulse.
Prescription: *Bai Ying* 30 g, *Long Kui* 20 g, *She Mei* 15 g, *Teng Li Gen* 15 g, *Bai Zhu* 10 g, *Fu Ling* 10 g, *Tu Fu Ling* 15 g, *Cao He Che* 15 g, *Sheng Huang Qi* 30 g, *Tai Zi Shen* 30 g, *Nü Zhen Zi* 15 g, *Gou Qi Zi* 10 g, *Jiao San Xian* 10 g each, *Sha Ren* 10 g and *Jiang Huang* 12 g.

Subsequent visit: 6 December 2002
The patient's condition was stable.
Prescription: *Bai Ying* 30 g, *Long Kui* 20 g, *She Mei* 15 g, *Teng Li Gen* 15 g, *Bai Zhu* 10 g, *Fu Ling* 10 g, *Tu Fu Ling* 15 g, *Cao He Che* 15 g, *Yuan Hu* 15 g, *Jiang Huang* 12 g, *Dong Ling Cao* 15 g, *Tai Zi Shen* 15 g, *Sheng Huang Qi* 30 g, *Nü Zhen Zi* 15 g, *Gou Qi Zi* 10 g, *Jiao San Xian* 10 g each and *Sha Ren* 10 g.

Date of visit: 18 April 2003
The patient did not show any obvious symptoms; condition was stable.
Prescription: *Teng Li Gen* 15 g, *Bai Ying* 30 g, *Long Kui* 15 g, *She Mei* 15 g, *Dong Ling Cao* 15 g, *Tu Fu Ling* 15 g, *Ba Yue Zha* 15 g,

Yuan Hu 15 g, *Zhong Jie Feng* 15 g, *Cao He Che* 15 g, *Sheng Huang Qi* 30 g, *Jiao San Xian* 30 g each, *Ji Nei Jin* 10 g and *Sha Ren* 10 g.

Date of visit: 27 June 2003
Cardiac carcinoma had been diagnosed for one and a half years. The patient now had no difficulty swallowing and enjoyed normal appetite, urination and bowel movements.
Prescription: Sheng Huang Qi 30 g, *Tai Zi Shen* 30 g, *Ji Xue Teng* 30 g, *Nü Zhen Zi* 15 g, *Gou Qi Zi* 10 g, *Teng Li Gen* 15 g, *Bai Ying* 30 g, *Long Kui* 15 g, *She Mei* 15 g, *Dong Ling Cao* 15 g, *Tu Fu Ling* 15 g, *Zhong Jie Feng* 15 g, *Ba Yue Zha* 15 g, *Jiao San Xian* 10 g each, *Ji Nei Jin* 10 g and *Sha Ren* 10 g.

Date of visit: 26 September 2003
The patient's general condition was still stable; cellular immune function was normal. The tongue was deep red with yellow fur, the pulse thready, taut and slippery.
Prescription: Sha Ren 30 g, *Tai Zi Shen* 30 g, *Sheng Huang Qi* 30 g, *Nü Zhen Zi* 15 g, *Gou Qi Zi* 10 g, *Zhi Qiao* 10 g, *Jiang Huang* 10 g, *Bai Ying* 30 g, *Long Kui* 15 g, *Tu Fu Ling* 15 g, *Ban Zhi Lian* 15 g, *Jiao San Xian* 10 g each, *Ji Nei Jin* 10 g, *Sha Ren* 10 g, *Sheng Gan Cao* 6 g and *Shi Hu* 10 g.

Date of visit: 4 November 2004
Gastroscopic examination showed a neoplasm at the lower cardiac corner, its border ulcerated and indistinct. The diagnosis was cardiac carcinoma (Borrmann type I). The patient insisted on continuing with herbal therapy.

Date of visit: 14 July 2006
Four and a half years after exploratory surgery, the patient's condition was stable and he generally felt well. He had a

good appetite and was in good spirits. Urination and bowel movements were normal; the tongue continued to be dark red with thin white fur; the pulse was taut, thready and slippery.

Prescription: *Sheng Huang Qi* 30 g, *Tai Zi Shen* 30 g, *Ji Xue Teng* 30 g, *Nü Zhen Zi* 15 g, *Gou Qi Zi* 10 g, *Jiang Huang* 10 g, *Bai Ying* 30 g, *Tu Fu Ling* 15 g, *Ban Zhi Lian* 15 g, *Teng Li Gen* 20 g, *Dong Ling Cao* 15 g, *Zhong Jie Feng* 15 g, *Ba Yue Zha* 15 g, *Jiao San Xian* 30 g each, *Ji Nei Jin* 10 g and *Sha Ren* 10 g.

Comments

1. Surgery for cardiac carcinoma was terminated because of a sharp drop in the patient's blood pressure. Because of the advanced age of the patient, radiotherapy and chemotherapy were also not used. Three days after surgery, he sought Chinese medical treatment. Based on the principle of increasing healthy *qi* and combating pathogenic factors, we adopted herbs that reinforced the spleen to increase healthy *qi*, like *Sheng Huang Qi*, *Tai Zi Shen*, *Nü Zhen Zi*, *Gou Qi Zi*, *Bai Zhu* and *Fu Ling*. These can strengthen the patient's immune function and resistance to disease. Herbs for detoxification and resisting cancer were added, including *Bai Ying*, *Long Kui*, *She Mei*, *Teng Li Gen*, *Tu Fu Ling*, *Cao He Che* and *Bai Hua She She Cao*. Herbs like *Xiao Ye Jin Qian Cao*, *Jiang Huang* and *Ji Xue Teng* were used for soothing the liver and gallbladder; and herbs like *Jiao San Xian*, *Ji Nei Jin* and *Sha Ren* for improving motility and appetite.

2. A significant feature of the case was that the Chinese medical herbs regulated the disorders induced by the cancer and

helped rebuild a new internal balance between healthy *qi* and pathogenic factors. It enabled the patient to *co-exist* with the cancer in his body, restraining its development and spread in order to prolong and enhance his quality of life. It illustrates how Chinese medical herbs can play an important role in the management of malignant tumours by encouraging internal balance in a terminally ill cancer patient.

Case 2

Female, 67 years old, artist.

First visit: 13 March 1998
Chief complaint: Three years after the gastric cancer operation, the patient suffered from tinnitus, acid regurgitation, thirst, constipation and insomnia.
History of present illness: Cancer resection three years ago; pathological examination showed adenocarcinoma with no lymph node metastasis; depth of infiltration unclear. Chemotherapy was administered after the operation. Recent examination did not reveal any significant abnormality other than gallstones and bile duct distension.
Current symptoms: Tongue red with little fur coating; pulse deep, thready and taut; tinnitus; constipation; insomnia; and thirst.
TCM syndrome differentiation: Yin deficiency and stagnation of liver *qi.*
Therapeutic principle: Soothing liver *qi* and nourishing stomach *yin.*
Prescription: Da Xiao Jin Qian Cao 30 g each, *Jiang Huang* 12 g, *Hu Zhang* 15 g, *Yu Jin* 10 g, *Ban Zhi Lian* 30 g, *Bai Hua She She*

Cao 30 g, *Sheng Huang Qi* 20 g, *Zhi Qiao* 10 g, *Shi Hu* 10 g, *Bei Sha Shen* 30 g, *Mai Dong* 15 g, *Nü Zhen Zi* 15 g, *Wu Wei Zi* 10 g and *Jiao San Xian* 10 g each.

Subsequent visit: 8 May 1998
Recent gastroscopy revealed ulcerative anastomotic stoma with mild gastric inflammation. The patient had poor sleep, fair appetite, occasional gastric discomfort and thirst. The tongue was deep red with no fur; the pulse deep, thready and weak.
Prescription: Sha Shen 30 g, *Mai Dong* 15 g, *Shi Hu* 15 g, *Tian Hua Fen* 15 g, *Sha Ren* 10 g, *Ji Nei Jin* 10 g, *Chuan Bei* 10 g, *Shan Zha* 10 g, *Cao He Che* 15 g, *Bai Hua She She Cao* 30 g, *Ban Zhi Lian* 20 g, *Hang Shao* 15 g, *Nü Zhen Zi* 15 g, *Sheng Huang Qi* 20 g and *Zhi Gan Cao* 6 g.

Date of visit: 5 June 1998
The symptoms were occasional stomach pain, fair appetite, occasional abdominal distension, dry stools one to two times a day, dry mouth, belching, good sleep, occasional anxiety attacks, yellow urine, blurring of vision, pain around the eyes; the tongue was dark with scanty fur; the pulse thready and slippery.
Prescription: Sha Shen 30 g, *Mai Dong* 15 g, *Wu Wei Zi* 10 g, *Tian Hua Fen* 15 g, *Sha Ren* 10 g, *Ji Nei Jin* 10 g, *Jiao San Xian* 10 g each, *Ji Xue Teng* 30 g, *Nü Zhen Zi* 12 g, *Gou Qi Zi* 10 g, *Hang Shao* 15 g, *Yuan Hu* 12 g, *Bai Hua She She Cao* 30 g, *Cao He Che* 15 g, *Sheng Huang Qi* 20 g and *Sheng Gan Cao* 4 g.

Date of visit: 20 August 1999
Four years after surgery, abdominal CT scan and blood picture showed no abnormality. The patient had occasional chest pain;

a red tongue with little fur; and a deep, thready and slippery pulse.

Prescription: *Sha Shen* 30 g, *Shi Hu* 15 g, *Mai Dong* 15 g, *Yu Zhu* 10 g, *Tian Hua Fen* 15 g, *Ji Xue Teng* 30 g, *Nü Zhen Zi* 15 g, *Gou Qi Zi* 10 g, *Bai Hua She She Cao* 30 g, *Hang Shao* 15 g, *Sheng Gan Cao* 6 g, *Teng Li Gen* 30 g, *Ban Zhi Lian* 20 g, *Sheng Huang Qi* 30 g and *Jiao San Xian* 10 g each.

In the subsequent six years, there were further visits each year; in general, the patient's condition was stable with no indication of a recurrence of cancer symptoms.

Date of visit: 22 April 2005
Nearly ten years after surgery for stomach cancer, the patient was in satisfactory condition with no sign of any spread of the cancer. Ultrasound scan revealed that the gallstones were still there. The patient's symptoms included thirst, gastric reflux, fair appetite, dry stools, normal vision, a dark tongue with little fur, and a deep, thready and weak pulse.

Prescription: *Sha Shen* 30 g, *Tai Zi Shen* 30 g, *Mai Dong* 15 g, *Tian Hua Fen* 15 g, *Shi Hu* 15 g, *E Zhu* 10 g, *Hu Zhang* 15 g, *Teng Li Gen* 30 g, *Nü Zhen Zi* 15 g, *Yu Zhu* 10 g, *Jiao San Xian* 10 g each, *Ji Nei Jin* 10 g, *Sha Ren* 10 g, *Cao Jue Ming* 15 g and *Yin Chen* 12 g.

Comments

1. Three years after surgery, although there was no recurrence of the cancer, the patient showed signs of severe damage to the stomach *yin* and gastric inflammation, consistent with deficiency of *qi* and *yin*, with symptoms of thirst, a red tongue with scanty fur, dry stools and dyspepsia. The use

of *Sha Shen, Mai Dong, Shi Hu, Tian Hua Fen, Yu Zhu* and *Hang Shao* addressed the problem by nourishing *yin* and promoting secretions of clear fluids.

2. The patient's gallstones and gastric inflammations could have caused pains in the chest region.

3. The decoctions used also contained smaller amounts of anti-cancer herbs like *Ban Zhi Lian, Bai Hua She She Cao, Hu Zhang, Bai Ying* and *Teng Li Gen* which could have helped prevent recurrence of the cancer. At 75 and after eight years of taking TCM decoctions, the patient was in satisfactory health and good spirits.

CHAPTER 6

DIET, EXERCISE AND HEALTH CULTIVATION

For the prevention of cancer, as well as for patients who have already contracted the illness, diet, exercise and the cultivation of health are of paramount importance. TCM looks at the human body holistically and regards cancers as originating from imbalance disorders in the body brought about by physical as well as emotional factors. This accounts for the critical roles that diet, exercise and health cultivation, including cultivation of the spirit, play in the management of cancer.

6.1. Nutrition in Cancer Prevention

Western medical science has a voluminous literature on the role of nutrition in the prevention of cancer as well as predisposing a person to cancer. However, many of these findings, including those from extensive clinical trials, are controversial and inconclusive. Most nutritionists recognize that foods that produce free radicals in our bodies predispose us to disease, including cancer. Free radicals are harmful chemical substances that induce metabolic injuries that accumulate over time and eventually cause disease. Advocates of diets rich in plants and grains and low in oils and animal products believe that plants and grains do not induce the "deadly cascade of free radicals" that assault the delicate membranes of cells; instead they contain antioxidants which help to neutralize free radicals and may help to prevent cancers, particularly cancers of the breast, prostate, colon, rectum, uterus and ovaries.[1]

The most comprehensive study of the role of diet in causing and preventing cancer is arguably that conducted by Colin Campbell when he was at Cornell University's Division of Nutritional Science.[2] Based on a 20-year epidemiological study of the dietary habits in 2400 counties in different regions of China and the incidence of serious diseases like cancer, coronary heart disease, stroke and diabetes, Campbell concluded that the ingestion of animal proteins is a strong predisposing factor towards these diseases, including cancer. A striking example is that of liver cancer associated with a fungus-produced toxin, aflatoxin, found in mouldy peanuts. Campbell's studies showed that children who had a high content of peanuts in their diet had higher rates of liver cancer. More significantly, children from wealthier families who consumed a high level of animal proteins had a higher rate of liver cancer than children who ate less animal protein and consumed more peanuts.

There is also extensive evidence suggesting that carcinogens found in some pesticides, food additives, and even food wrappers and containers contribute significantly to the incidence of certain cancers. In addition, various nutritionists have long lists of healthy foods that they claim reduce the incidence of cancer; many of these are ordinary vegetables like broccoli, tomatoes and garlic. This subject will undoubtedly continue to engage the efforts of nutritional research scientists the world over.

---

[1] See Esselstyn (2008), pp. 38, 108.
[2] Campbell and Campbell (2007).

6.2. Nutritional Therapy for Cancer Patients

Cancer is a systemic disease. It is characterized not only by localized progressive uncontrolled growth and its ability to infiltrate and destroy normal tissues and organs, but also by a series of nutritional and metabolic problems that could leave the patient debilitated and emaciated, eventually resulting in organ failure and death.

There are several factors that contribute to nutritional disorders in cancer patients. The first factor is reduced food intake and absorption, which is attributed to the production of toxins from tumour metabolism. Consequently, symptoms such as loss of appetite and weight loss are observed in the initial stage of cancer. The second factor arises from the body being deprived of nutrients because of the rapid growth of cancer cells. When the patient receives treatments such as chemotherapy, radiotherapy and surgical interventions, further damage is inflicted. Nausea, bloating of the abdomen and difficulty ingesting food are some of the more common side effects of such therapy, leading to a further deterioration in nutritional health.

The importance of nutritional problems is often overlooked by both doctors and patients. There is a tendency for doctors to focus more on the efficacy of the treatment in combating cancer cells and neglecting the harmful effects of nutritional deficiencies. This can be exacerbated by lack of knowledge and guidance in nutrition on the part of the patient and his supporting family, thus leading to the consumption of large amounts of foods that are unsuitable for the patient's condition and aggravate the impairment of his digestive system.

Inappropriate nutrition for cancer patients can have adverse clinical consequences. Hence, it is necessary to use the correct diet and to improve the patient's medical condition to give him the best chance of controlling the progression of the disease.

Certain guidelines should be followed in planning nutrition for cancer patients:

1. It is essential to conduct an assessment of the nutritional status of the patient before and during the course of treatment to help decide the diet and supplemental nutrients required by the patient. Nutritional therapy can improve the patient's immune system, helping the body to better cope with the side effects of cancer treatments. Hence, nutritional therapy should be included in all cancer patients' personalized treatment plan.

2. Nutritional therapy should start early. The choice of nutritional therapy is dependent on several factors, such as the cause of nutrition disorder, the progression of the disease, the side effects of cancer treatments, the psychological state of the patient, as well as economical and social issues.

3. The mode of administration for late-stage cancer patients should be one that is life-supporting, be it short-term or long-term. Examples of these modes of administration are oral, nasal and parenteral (i.e. not through the mouth).

4. The effect of nutrition on cancer cell growth and the patient's ability to resist the disease has been a matter of controversy. One point of view is that nutrition to maintain body weight can encourage the growth of cancer cells. Some animal studies seem to suggest that improving the nutritional health status of the patient can increase the growth rate and size of cancer cells but other studies indicate that such an outcome is rare. Experiments on mice have demonstrated that there is no change in the uncontrolled growth rate of metastasized cancerous cells even when they are injected with large amount of nutrients. Nevertheless, in a situation when cancer cells are present during the course of nutritional therapy, it is

essential to include other forms of treatment aimed at controlling cancer cell growth.

5. An important and primary objective of nutritional therapy is to increase the body's ability to assimilate and metabolize food intake. TCM methods can be quite effective toward this end.

6.3. TCM Perspectives of Appropriate Diets for Cancer Patients

Despite a wealth of knowledge on nutrition in Chinese medicine accumulated from ancient times, further intensive research should be conducted using modern nutritional knowledge to understand and assess TCM dietary practices and perspectives. With particular reference to cancer patients, a number of dietary principles are worthy of note:

1. To prevent the recurrence of cancer, one should avoid eating food that is mouldy, deep-fried, stale, high in glucose or contains nitrosamines.
2. In TCM theory, the spleen and stomach are responsible for the digestion and absorption of nutrients essential to health. Hence, emphasis is placed on the importance of protecting the spleen and stomach, especially when patients are under-going chemotherapy, radiotherapy as well as TCM treat-ments. Foods that will harm the digestive system should be avoided.
3. Cancer patients are often depressed and worried over their conditions. Such emotional states can damage the functions of the spleen and stomach, resulting in loss of appetite and reduced food intake and adversely affecting the efficacy of

cancer treatments. Establishing a good physician-patient
relationship helps the patient to have more confidence and
adopt a more optimistic attitude. This in turn leads to an
improvement in the absorption and metabolism of the nutrients by the body and a better prospect for improvement in
the patient's condition or recovery.

4. In Chinese medicine, food can be classified according to five
    flavours and four natures. The five flavours are pungent,
    sweet, sour, bitter and salty, and the four natures are cold, hot,
    warm and cool. As pointed out in Chapter 2 of this book, the
    core approach of TCM diagnosis and treatment lies in syn-
    drome differentiation. As a broad principle, the type of diet
    for cancer patients should therefore be based on the syn-
    drome presented. For every type and stage of disease, differ-
    ent patients present different syndromes. For example,
    patients who present hot syndrome should avoid foods that
    are warm in nature, such as ginseng, venison, lamb, longan
    and prawn, and are better off eating foods that are cool in
    nature and have the functions of clearing heat and reducing
    inflammation, such as purslane, lotus, asparagus and duck.
    Some people advocate cancer patients eating Chinese soft-
    shell turtle, but one should be aware that turtle cools the
    blood and nourishes *yin*, and is also harder to digest. It is not
    suitable for patients who exhibit spleen and *yang* deficiency.
    Hence, the syndrome presented by the patient is the most
    suitable determinant of the appropriate foods for his diet.

5. Another class of foods that should be given to the patient is
    those that strengthen healthy *qi* and/or have anti-cancer
    properties. A variety of cereals, meat, fruits and vegetables
    can strengthen healthy *qi*. If the patient's spleen and stom-
    ach are functioning satisfactorily, foods thought to have
    anti-cancer properties like shepherd's purse (荠菜),

Chinese barley (Job's tears 生苡米), purslane (马齿苋), *Doellingeria scaber* (东风菜), *Isoden* (香茶菜), bitter gourd, day lily (黄花菜), warrigal greens (番杏), walnut, seaweed, water chestnut (荸荠), caltrop (菱角) and mushroom may be suitable.

A list of common foods with anti-cancer effects is provided in Appendix 2.

6.4. Dietary Restrictions

Diet has a close relationship to the occurrence and development of cancerous tumours, hence it is essential to consider dietary restrictions for cancer patients. However, although many ancient Chinese medical texts advise strict control over the diets of sick patients, from the point of view of the modern understanding of nutrition they may be overly restrictive.

Over several decades of medical practice, I have come across many patients who, despite having undergone surgery, chemotherapy or radiotherapy, do not observe dietary restrictions, eating such diverse foods as chicken, fish, prawns, sea cucumber, lamb, venison and even dog meat. But there was little evidence that they had cancer relapses on account of such diets. There is also a belief in some quarters that eating chicken can cause cancer. But Chinese medical records suggest that chicken helps the body overcome deficiency syndromes and recover from post-illness weakness, warms the middle interior, and strengthens the five *zang* organs. In fact some folk recipes for cancer have a combination of chicken eggs with twigs of the walnut tree or Chinese blister beetle (*Cantharis* or Spanish fly). Many cancer patients eat chicken with no evidence that it is harmful to their condition. Sea cucumber has been found from modern research to have anti-cancer properties.

Our considered opinion is that diet should be suited to the individual person and his particular medical condition at a particular time and we should avoid making vague generalized statements about what can or cannot be consumed by cancer patients. Although we respect ancient advice on this matter, it is also necessary to avoid going overboard and placing unnecessary restrictions on the diet of cancer patients. Professor Yu has personally witnessed patients who, following prohibitions on a number of common foodstuffs such as bean curd, eggs and vegetables in their diet, ended up with inadequate nutrition, which worked against their process of recovery. Our conclusion is that diets should not be too strict or restricted, and that close attention should be paid to the condition of the patient's spleen and stomach, whether it is assimilating food well or showing syndromes of cold, heat, deficiency or excess. Only then can he get the best benefit from the therapies he is receiving.

As a general guideline, a cancer patient at the beginning of treatment need not have dietary restrictions. Instead he should try a small quantity of each kind of food. He would know after some time what kind of food agrees with him, based on the reaction of his digestive system to it and the presence or otherwise of any side effects of consuming the food. He should avoid food that does not agree with him and continue to eat food that he finds he can digest well and agrees with his body.

6.5. Exercise and Life Cultivation

Qigong is one of the treasures of Chinese medical wisdom. From the point of view of traditional Chinese medicine, the enhancement of *qi* within one's own body through *qigong* exercises is a positive factor in cancer prevention and treatment. This observation applies to exercises practised on one's own body through breathing and physical movement. Concerning claims of *qigong* healing by transferring "*qi*" from the healer to the patient, we believe that the psychological factor and the placebo effect could be relevant, but are not aware of clinical trials that conclusively demonstrate therapeutic effects.

Based on Professor Yu's clinical experience, we believe *qigong*'s benefit to the human body works in the following ways:

1. *Qigong* assists in the flow of *qi* and blood. This is beneficial to cancer patients as a common condition accompanying this disease is stagnation of *qi* and blood stasis.
2. *Qigong* helps regulate the functions of internal organs, in particular digestive functions, breathing, and circulatory and neurological functions.
3. The mind is focused on the *dantian* in the lower abdominal region during *qigong* meditation. This helps the mind dispel negative thoughts and anxiety, helps the patient develop more self-confidence, and has a calming psychological effect on the patient which helps with his recovery.
4. *Qigong* exercises can help strengthen the immune system of the patient, assisting him to cope with his condition and possibly helping in his recovery.

In the lung cancer section in the last chapter, we mentioned the case of a patient who survived for 23 years after contracting late-stage lung cancer. We believe that his practice of *qigong* together with the use of Chinese herbal medications played a large role in his recovery.

Health preservation is but a major aspect of the wider concept of *yangsheng* or the cultivation of life. The medical classic *Huangdi neijing* laid down the basic rules of life cultivation that promotes longevity and helps prevent disease, including cancer.

These rules are also applicable to those who have already contracted cancer, by improving the quality of life and reducing the chances of relapse.

A celebrated passage from the *Neijing* on life cultivation is worth citing here:

> The ancients knew the *tao* and understood the way of *yin* and *yang*, and how to exercise; moderation in food and drink, regularity in living habits, avoidance of overexertion, maintaining harmony between body and spirit.[3]

To know the *tao* and the way of *yin* and *yang* is to be able to go with the flow of nature and to achieve balance with the external environment and within the body as well. Exercise involves breathing as in *qigong* meditation and movement as in *taiji* and similar exercises. Moderation in food and drink involves observing good dietary habits and eating regular meals without excessive consumption of food and alcohol. Regularity in living habits would ideally follow the cycle of day and night, sleeping earlier in winter months when the sun sets early and rising early in summer months. Exercise and meals should be at fixed times and regular working hours observed rather than burning the midnight oil to complete urgent tasks. Overexertion, a problem endemic in busy cities like Beijing, London and Singapore, harms the body's *yuan qi*, and emotional factors associated with stress damage our vital organs. Excessive sexual indulgence also depletes *jing* and *qi* in the body and harms the kidney functions. Most important of all, maintaining a relaxed mind in harmony with the body is our best insurance against long-term ailments that develop insidiously in our bodies.

---

[3] The original Chinese text reads "上古之人，其知道者：法于阴阳，和与术数，饮食有节，起居有常：不妄作劳，故能形与神俱". See *Yellow Emperor's Canon of Medicine* (2005).

The *Neijing* has another famous passage that elaborates on avoidance of illness:

> Know when to avoid climatic stresses, live a placid life with plain needs, maintain the defensive forces in your body, stay in good spirits. When you do all this, how then could you possibly fall ill?[4]

This passage draws on the theory of TCM that attributes the fundamental causes of illness to climatic and emotional factors that we described in Chapter 2. Exposure to extremes of heat or cold, humidity, wind and dryness can cause harmful pathogens to invade our bodies and, if not repelled in good time, transform into internal pathogenic factors that bring about changing syndromes that become more entrenched with time if not treated and managed properly.

The *Neijing* here again emphasizes the importance of the mind, or spirit, in preventing illness and maintaining good health. This is achieved not just by avoiding and managing emotional stress, but also by engaging in activities that elevate the spirit and nourish the soul. In Chinese tradition, engagement in chess games, music (such as playing stringed instruments like the *qin*), painting and calligraphy and the enjoyment of poetry are forms of *yangsheng*, or the cultivation of life. *Yangsheng* is holistic. It requires us to cultivate the body through diet and exercise, regularity in living habits and avoidance of external pathogens, but also to cultivate the mind through relaxing and enjoyable activities. Such a holistic approach to life is our best defence against illness and gives us the best chance of avoiding the development of cancer cells in the body.

---

[4] 虚邪贼风，避之有时，恬淡虚无，真气从之，精神内守，病安从来.

REFERENCES

Campbell TC and Campbell TM. (2007) *The China Study*, Ben Bella Books, Dallas.

Chai K. (ed.) (2007) *Fundamental Theory of Traditional Chinese Medicine*, People's Medical Publishing Home, Beijing.

Esselystyn CB. (2008) *Prevent and Reverse Heart Disease*, Avery, New York.

Farquhar J. (1994) *Knowing Practice: The Clinical Encounter in Chinese Medicine*, Westview Press, Boulder, CO.

Hong H. (2009) Kuhn and the two cultures of Chinese and Western medicine. Journal of Cambridge Studies, Vol. 4, No. 3, pp. 10–36. Association of Cambridge Studies, Cambridge, UK.

Kuriyama S. (1999) *The Expressiveness of the Body*, Zone Books, New York.

Lei S. (1999) *When Chinese Medicine Encountered the State, 1910–1949*, PhD dissertation, University of Chicago.

Neese RM and Williams GC. (1996) *Why We Get Sick: The New Science of Darwinian Medicine*, Vintage Books, New York.

Ou J. (2005) *Dang Zhongyi Yushang Xiyi* 当中医遇上西医 (*When Chinese Medicine Meets Western Medicine*), Sanlian Shudian, Hong Kong.

Oxford Concise Medical Dictionary, 4th Edition. (2007) Oxford University Press.

Scheid V. (2002) *Chinese Medicine in Contemporary China: Plurality and Synthesis*, Duke University Press, Durham, NC.

Schwartz V. (1986) The enduring challenge of enlightenment, in *The Chinese Enlightenment*, University of California Press, Berkeley, CA, pp. 283–302.

Sivin N. (1987) *Traditional Medicine in Contemporary China*, University of Michigan Press, Ann Arbor, MI.

Taylor K. (2005) *Chinese Medicine in Early Communist China, 1945–1963*, Routledge Curzon, New York.

Unschuld P. (2003) *Huang Di Nei Jing Su Wen: Nature, Knowledge, Imagery in an Ancient Chinese Medical Text*, University of California Press, Berkeley, CA.

Wang X. (ed.) (2001) *Zhongyi Jichu Lilun* 中医基础理论, *Renmin Weisheng Chubanshe*, Beijing, p. 44.

Wu C. (ed.) (2002) *Basic Theory of Traditional Chinese Medicine*, Shanghai University of TCM Publishing House, Shanghai (in Chinese with English translation).

Yellow Emperor's Canon of Medicine 黄帝内经. (2005) Xian World Publishing Company.

Yu R, *et al.* (2007) *Yu Rencun* 郁仁存, Zhongguo Zhongyiyao Chuban She, Beijing.

HERBS USED IN CANCER THERAPY

For your easy reference, we have compiled in Table A.1 the herbs used for cancer therapy that have been mentioned in the book. Most herbs have several therapeutic effects although only one or two of these effects may be used within each prescription for a specific condition.

Note: The term "sheng" (生) in front of the name of a herb indicates that it is used in raw unprocessed form; "jiao" (焦) indicates that it has been charred by a frying process. "Parched" also indicates that the herb has undergone the process of frying (炒) to enhance its effects for fortifying the spleen and strengthening qi.

Table A.1.   Herbs Used for Cancer Therapy.

Name in *Pinyin*	Chinese Name	Latin Name	Common Name	Therapeutic Functions
Ai Ye	艾叶	*Folium Artemisiae Argyi*	Argy Wormwood Leaf	1. Warms the meridians and expels cold 2. Stops bleeding 3. Regulates the menstrual cycle 4. Prevents miscarriage
Ba Yue Zha/Yu Zhi Zi	八月札/预知子	*Fructus Akebiae*	Akebia Fruit	1. Disperses stagnation of liver *qi* 2. Regulates the stomach functions 3. Improves blood circulation to relieve pain 4. Softens and disperses masses/abnormal growth 5. Promotes diuresis
Bai Bu	百部	*Radix Stemonae*	Sessile Stemona Root/Japanese Stemona Root/Tuber Stemona	1. Nourishes the lung and relieves cough 2. Kills parasites
Bai He	百合	*Bulbus Lilii*	Lanceleaf Lily Bulb/Greenish Lily Bulb/Low Lily Bulb	1. Nourishes *yin* and moistens the lung 2. Clears heart heat and calms the mind
Bai Hua She She Cao	白花蛇舌草	*Herba Hedyotidis Diffusae*	Spreading Hedyotis Herb	1. Anti-inflammatory effect 2. Removes dampness and promote diuresis

(*Continued*)

Table A.1. (*Continued*).

Name in *Pinyin*	Chinese Name	Latin Name	Common Name	Therapeutic Functions
Bai Kou Ren/Bai Dou Kou	白寇仁/白豆蔻	*Fructus Amomi Rotundus*	Round Cardamom Fruit/Java Amomum Fruit	1. Removes dampness and relieves *qi* stagnation in the abdomen 2. Warms the abdomen 3. Relieves nausea and vomiting (anti-emetic effect)
Bai Shao/Hang Shao/Hanzhou Bai Shao	白芍/杭芍	*Radix Paeoniae Alba*	White Peony Root	1. Nourishes the blood 2. Retains *yin* 3. Soothes the liver and relieves pain 4. Stops excessive perspiration
Bai Tou Weng	白头翁	*Radix Pulsatillae*	Chinese Pulsatilla Root	1. Anti-inflammatory effect 2. Cools the blood and treats dysentery
Bai Xian Pi	白鲜皮	*Cortex Dictamni*	Densefruit Pittany Root-bark	1. Removes damp-heat 2. Expels wind 3. Detoxification effect
Bai Ying	白英	*Herba Solani Lyrati*	Bittersweet Herb	1. Clears heat and removes dampness 2. Detoxification 3. Reduces swelling 4. Anti-cancer effect

(*Continued*)

Table A.1. (*Continued*).

Name in *Pinyin*	Chinese Name	Latin Name	Common Name	Therapeutic Functions
Bai Zhi	白芷	*Radix Angelicae Dahuricae*	Dahurian Angelica Root/ Taiwan Angelica Root	1. Expels cold and wind to relieve pain 2. Clears the nasal passages to alleviate blocked nose 3. Stops abnormal vaginal discharges (leucorrhoea) by removing dampness 4. Reduces swelling of wounds 5. Eliminates pus
Bai Zhu	白术	*Rhizoma Atractylodis Macrocephalae*	Largehead Atractylodes Rhizome	1. Fortifies the spleen and strengthens *qi* 2. Promotes diuresis by removing dampness 3. Stops perspiration (anhidrotic effect)
Bai Zi Ren	柏子仁	*Semen Platycladi*	Chinese Arborvitae Kernel	1. Clears heart heat and calms the mind 2. Stimulates bowel movement
Ban Bian Lian	半边莲	*Herba Lobeliae Chinensis*	Chinese Lobelia Herb	1. Anti-inflammatory effect 2. Reduces oedema
Ban Mao	斑蝥	*Mylabris*	Blister Beetle	1. Strong effect on improving blood circulation and removing blood stasis 2. Counteract toxins to promote wound/ ulcer/carbuncle healing

(Continued)

Table A.1. (*Continued*).

Name in *Pinyin*	Chinese Name	Latin Name	Common Name	Therapeutic Functions
Ban Xia	半夏	*Rhizoma Pinelliae*	Pinellia Tuber	1. Resolves dampness and phlegm 2. Relieves nausea and vomiting 3. Relieves stagnation and disperses masses/abnormal growth
Ban Zhi Lian	半枝莲	*Herba Scutellariae Barbatae*	Barbed Skullcap Herb	1. Anti-inflammatory effect 2. Stops bleeding by removing blood stasis 3. Relieves oedema
Bei Dou Gen	北豆根	*Rhizoma Menispermi*	Asiatic Moonseed Rhizome	1. Anti-inflammatory effect 2. Expels wind 3. Relieves pain
Bei Sha Shen	北沙参	*Radix Glehniae*	Coastal Glehnia Root	1. Nourishes *yin* and clears lung heat 2. Strengthens the stomach functions 3. Promotes the production of body fluids
Bie Jia Jiao	鳖甲胶	*Colla Carapacis Trionycis*	Turtle Shell Glue	1. Nourishes *yin* 2. Anti-pyretic effect 3. Softens and disperses masses/abnormal growth

(*Continued*)

Table A.1. (*Continued*).

Name in *Pinyin*	Chinese Name	Latin Name	Common Name	Therapeutic Functions
Bu Gu Zhi	补骨脂	*Fructus Psoraleae*	Malaytea Scurfpea Fruit	1. Tonifies the kidney and strengthens *yang* 2. Consolidates essence to treat enuresis and involuntary seminal emission 3. Warms the spleen to relieve diarrhoea 4. Anti-asthmatic effect
Cang Zhu	苍术	*Rhizoma Atractylodis*	Swordlike Atractylodes Rhizome/Chinese Atractylodes Rhizome	1. Removes dampness 2. Strengthens the spleen functions 3. Expels wind and cold
Cao He Che	草河车	*Rhizoma Paridis*	Yunnan Manyleaf Paris Rhizome/Chinese Paris Rhizome	1. Anti-inflammatory effect 2. Reduces swelling and relieves pain 3. Cools the liver to relieve convulsions
Cao Jue Ming	草决明	*Semen Cassiae*	Cassia Seed	1. Clears heat and improves vision 2. Promotes bowel movement
Chai Hu	柴胡	*Radix Bupleuri*	Chinese Thorowax Root/ Red Thorowax Root	1. Relieves exterior syndrome 2. Anti-pyretic effect 3. Disperses stagnation of liver *qi* 4. Uplifts *yang qi* to prevent the descent of *yang*

(*Continued*)

Table A.1.   (*Continued*).

Name in *Pinyin*	Chinese Name	Latin Name	Common Name	Therapeutic Functions
Che Qian Cao	车前草	*Herba Plantaginis*	Plantain Herb	1. Promotes diuresis 2. Relieves diarrhoea 3. Anti-inflammatory effect
Chen Pi/Ju Pi	陈皮 / 橘皮	*Pericarpium Citri Reticulatae*	Dried Tangerine Peel	1. Regulates *qi* in the abdomen and strengthens the spleen functions 2. Resolves dampness and phlegm
Chi Shao	赤芍	*Radix Paeoniae Rubra*	Red Peony Root	1. Removes heat in the blood 2. Dissipates blood stasis to relieve pain
Chou Chun Pi Gen	臭椿皮根	*Cortex Ailanthi*	Tree-of-heaven Ailanthus Bark	1. Clears heat and removes dampness 2. Induces astringency to treat abnormal vaginal discharges 3. Relieves diarrhoea 4. Stops bleeding
Chou Hu Lu	抽葫芦	*Fructus Lagenariae*	Bottle Gourd Peel	1. Relieves oedema
Chuan Bei Mu	川贝母	*Bulbus Fritillariae Unibracteatae*	Unibract Fritillary Bulb	1. Clears heat and resolves phlegm 2. Moistens the lung to relieve cough 3. Disperses masses/abnormal growth and reduces carbuncle swelling

(Continued)

Table A.1. (*Continued*).

Name in *Pinyin*	Chinese Name	Latin Name	Common Name	Therapeutic Functions
Chuan Lian Zi	川楝子	*Fructus Toosendan*	Szechwan Chinaberry Fruit	1. Promotes the flow of *qi* 2. Relieves pain 3. Kills parasites
Chang Pu	菖蒲	*Rhizoma Atractylodis*	Grassleaf Sweetflag Rhizome	1. Restores consciousness 2. Removes dampness and regulates the stomach functions 3. Calms the nerves and mind 4. Improves intelligence
Chuan Shan Jia	穿山甲	*Squama Manitis*	Pangolin Scales	1. Improves blood circulation and disperses masses/abnormal growth 2. Stimulates menstruation 3. Promotes lactation 4. Reduces swelling and induces pus discharge of wounds/ulcers/carbuncles
Chuan Xiong	川芎	*Rhizoma Ligustici Chuanxiong*	Szechwan Lovage Rhizome	1. Improves blood circulation 2. Promotes the flow of *qi* 3. Expels wind 4. Relieves pain

(*Continued*)

Table A.1. (*Continued*).

Name in *Pinyin*	Chinese Name	Latin Name	Common Name	Therapeutic Functions
Ci Wu Jia	刺五加	*Radix Acanthopanacis Senticosi*	Manyprickle Acanto-Panax Root	1. Fortifies the spleen and strengthens *qi* 2. Tonifies the kidney 3. Calms the nerves and mind
Da Fu Pi	大腹皮	*Pericarpium Arecae*	Areca Peel	1. Promotes the flow of *qi* to relieve *qi* stagnation in the abdomen 2. Reduces oedema
Da Huang	大黄	*Radix et Rhizoma Rhei*	Rhubarb	1. Stimulates the bowel 2. Clears heat and purges fire 3. Cools the blood 4. Detoxification effects 5. Dissipates blood stasis to stimulate menstruation
Da Zao	大枣	*Fructus Jujubae*	Chinese Date	1. Tonifies the spleen and stomach functions and strengthens *qi* 2. Nourishes the blood 3. Calms the nerves and mind
Dai Zhe Shi	代赭石	*Ochre Haematitum*	Red Ochre/ Haematite	1. Suppresses liver *yang* 2. Promotes descent of *qi* 3. Cools the blood to stop bleeding

(*Continued*)

Table A.1. (*Continued*).

Name in *Pinyin*	Chinese Name	Latin Name	Common Name	Therapeutic Functions
Dan Pi	丹皮	*Cortex Moutan*	Tree Peony Bark	1. Removes heat in the blood 2. Improves blood circulation and removes blood stasis
Dan Nan Xing	胆南星	*Bile Arisaema*	Arisaema cum Bile	1. Clears heat and resolves phlegm 2. Subdues endogenous wind to relieve convulsions
Dan Shen	丹参	*Radix Salviae Miltiorrhizae*	Danshen Root	1. Improves blood circulation 2. Regulates menstruation 3. Removes blood stasis to relieve pain 4. Cools the blood 5. Promotes healing of carbuncles 6. Calms the mind
Dang Gui	当归	*Radix Angelicae Sinensis*	Chinese Angelica	1. Enriches the blood 2. Regulates menstruation 3. Improves blood circulation 4. Relieves pain 5. Stimulates bowel movement

(*Continued*)

Table A.1. (*Continued*).

Name in *Pinyin*	Chinese Name	Latin Name	Common Name	Therapeutic Functions
Dang Shen	党参	*Radix Codonopsis*	Pilose Asiabell Root/Moderate Asiabell Root/Szechwon Tangshen Root	1. Invigorates the spleen and lung functions 2. Enriches the blood 3. Promotes the production of body fluids
Di Fu Zi	地肤子	*Fructus Kochiae*	Belvedere Fruit	1. Promotes diuresis 2. Clears heat and removes dampness 3. Relieves itching
Dong Ling Cao	冬凌草	*Rabdosia Rubescens*	Blushred Rabdosia	1. Anti-inflammatory effect 2. Improves blood circulation to relieve pain
Du Zhong	杜仲	*Cortex Eucommiae*	Eucommia Bark	1. Tonifies the liver and kidney 2. Strengthens tendons and bones 3. Prevents miscarriage
E Jiao	阿胶	*Colla Corii Asini*	Donkey-hide Glue	1. Enriches the blood 2. Nourishes *yin* 3. Moistens the lung 4. Stops bleeding

(*Continued*)

Table A.1. (*Continued*).

Name in Pinyin	Chinese Name	Latin Name	Common Name	Therapeutic Functions
E Zhu	莪术	*Rhizoma Curcumae*	Zedoary	1. Strong effect on improving blood circulation 2. Promotes the flow of *qi* 3. Promotes digestion of residual food to relieve *qi* stagnation 4. Relieves pain
Fang Feng	防风	*Radix Saposhnikoviae*	Divaricate Saposhnikovia Root	1. Expels wind 2. Removes dampness 3. Relieves pain and convulsions
Feng Fang	蜂房	*Nidus Vespae*	Honeycomb	1. Counteracts toxins to kill parasites 2. Expels wind and relieves pain
Fu Ling/ Yun Ling	茯苓/云苓	*Poria*	Hoelen	1. Relieves oedema 2. Removes dampness 3. Strengthens the spleen 4. Calms the mind
Fu Pen Zi	覆盆子	*Fructus Rubi*	Palmleaf Raspberry Fruit	1. Consolidates essence to treat enuresis and involuntary seminal emission 2. Strengthens the liver and kidney functions 3. Improves vision

(*Continued*)

Table A.1. (*Continued*).

Name in *Pinyin*	Chinese Name	Latin Name	Common Name	Therapeutic Functions
Fu Rong Ye	芙蓉叶	*Folium Hibisci Mutabilis*	Cotton Rose Hibiscus Leaf	1. Clears lung heat 2. Cools the blood 3. Reduces swelling and induces pus discharge
Fu Rong Hua	芙蓉花	*Hibiscus mutabilis L.*	Cotton Rose Hibiscus Flower	1. Removes heat in the blood 2. Reduces swelling and induces pus discharge
Fu Xiao Mai	浮小麦	*Fructus Tritici Levis*	Blighted Wheat	1. Consolidates the exterior to stop perspiration 2. Strengthens *qi* 3. Clears heat
Gan Cao	甘草	*Radix Glycyrrhizae*	Liquorice Root	1. Fortifies the spleen and strengthens *qi* 2. Resolves phlegm and relieves cough 3. Relieves pain 4. Anti-inflammatory effect 5. Regulates the functions of herbs in the formula
Gang Ban Gui	杠板归	*Herba Polygoni Perfoliati*	Perfoliate Knotweed Herb	1. Relieves oedema and cough 2. Anti-inflammatory effect

(*Continued*)

Table A.1. (*Continued*).

Name in *Pinyin*	Chinese Name	Latin Name	Common Name	Therapeutic Functions
Gou Ju Li	枸橘李	*Poncirus Trifoliata*	Trifoliate-orange Immature Fruit	1. Disperses the stagnation of liver *qi* and regulates the stomach functions 2. Promotes the flow of *qi* to relieve pain 3. Promotes digestion to relieve *qi* stagnation in the abdomen
Gou Qi Zi	枸杞子	*Fructus Lycii*	Barbary Wolfberry Fruit	1. Nourishes the liver and kidney 2. Enriches the essence 3. Improves vision
Gua Lou	瓜蒌	*Fructus Trichosanthis*	Snakegourd Fruit	1. Clears heat and resolves phlegm 2. Relieves *qi* stagnation in the chest 3. Disperses masses 4. Stimulates bowel movement
Gui Ban Jiao	龟板胶	*Chinemys reevesii*	Tortoise Shell Glue	1. Nourishes *yin* and suppresses *yang* 2. Invigorates the kidney and strengthens bones 3. Enriches the blood 4. Stops bleeding

(*Continued*)

Table A.1. (*Continued*).

Name in *Pinyin*	Chinese Name	Latin Name	Common Name	Therapeutic Functions
Gui Jian Yu	鬼箭羽	*Ramulus Euonymi*	Winged Euonymus Twig	1. Strong effect on improving blood circulation 2. Stimulates menstruation 3. Detoxification effect 4. Reduces swelling 5. Kills parasites
Hai Zao	海藻	*Sargassum*	Seaweed	1. Resolves phlegm and softens the masses/abnormal growth 2. Relieves oedema
Han Lian Cao	旱莲草	*Herba Ecliptae*	Yerbadetajo Herb	1. Nourishes the liver and kidney 2. Cools the blood to stop bleeding
Hang Ju	杭菊	*Chrysanthemum morifolium*	Chrysanthemum Flower (from Hangzhou)	1. Expels exogenous wind-heat 2. Suppresses liver *yang* 3. Clears liver heat and improves vision 4. Anti-inflammatory effect
Hou Po/ Chuan Pu	厚朴/川朴	*Cortex Magnoliae Officinalis*	Officinal Magnolia Bark	1. Removes dampness and resolves phlegm 2. Relieves *qi* stagnation in the abdomen

(*Continued*)

Table A.1. (*Continued*).

Name in *Pinyin*	Chinese Name	Latin Name	Common Name	Therapeutic Functions
Hou Po Hua	厚朴花	*Flos Magnoliae Officinalis*	Official Magnolia Flower	1. Similar therapeutic effects to but generally milder than *Hou Po* (厚朴)
Hu Zhang	虎杖	*Rhizoma Polygoni Cuspidati*	Giant Knotweed Rhizome	1. Removes dampness to treat jaundice 2. Anti-inflammatory effect 3. Relieves pain by removing blood stasis 4. Relieves cough by resolving phlegm
Huang Bai	黄柏	*Cortex Phellodendri*	Amur Corktree Bark	1. Removes damp-heat 2. Purges fire 3. Promotes wound/ ulcer healing via detoxification *Note: Frying Huang Bai helps to reduce its cold nature, hence softening its effects of clearing heat and purging fire. This prevents damage to the spleen and stomach, and makes it suitable for individuals with weak or impaired digestive systems.*

(*Continued*)

Table A.1. (*Continued*).

Name in *Pinyin*	Chinese Name	Latin Name	Common Name	Therapeutic Functions
Huang Jing	黄精	*Rhizoma Polygonati*	Manyflower Solomonseal Rhizome/ Siberian Solomonseal Rhizome/King Solomonseal Rhizome	1. Invigorates *qi* and nourishes *yin* 2. Strengthens the spleen and kidney functions 3. Nourishes the lung
Huang Lian	黄连	*Rhizoma Coptidis*	Golden Thread	1. Removes damp-heat 2. Purges fire 3. Detoxification effect
Huang Qi	黄芪	*Radix Astragali*	Membranous Milkvetch Root/ Mongolian Milkvetch Root	1. Strengthens the spleen functions 2. Uplifts *yang qi* to prevent the descent of *yang* 3. Consolidates the exterior to strengthen the body's external defence 4. Promotes diuresis 5. Promotes healing of wounds/ulcers
Huang Qin	黄芩	*Radix Scutellariae*	Baical Skullcap Root	1. Removes damp-heat 2. Purges fire 3. Detoxification effect 4. Stops bleeding 5. Prevents miscarriages

(*Continued*)

Table A.1.   (*Continued*).

Name in *Pinyin*	Chinese Name	Latin Name	Common Name	Therapeutic Functions
Huo Xiang	藿香	*Herba Agastaches*	Wrinkled Gianthyssop Herb	1. Removes dampness 2. Relieves nausea and vomiting 3. Clears summer-heat
Ji Nei Jin	鸡内金	*Endothelium Corneum Gigeriae Galli*	Chicken's Gizzard-membrane	1. Promotes digestion 2. Strengthens the stomach functions 3. Induces astringency to treat enuresis and involuntary seminal emission
Ji Xue Teng	鸡血藤	*Caulis Spatholobi*	Suberect Spatholobus Stem	1. Enriches the blood and improves blood circulation 2. Regulates menstruation 3. Nourishes the tendons to improve limb movements
Jiang Can	僵蚕	*Bombyx Batryticatus*	Stiff Silkworm	1. Expels exogenous wind 2. Subdues endogenous to relieve convulsions 3. Resolves phlegm to disperse masses/abnormal growth

(*Continued*)

Table A.1. (*Continued*).

Name in *Pinyin*	Chinese Name	Latin Name	Common Name	Therapeutic Functions
Jiang Huang	姜黄	*Rhizoma Curcumae Longae*	Turmeric	1. Improves blood circulation 2. Promotes the flow of *qi* 3. Stimulates menstruation 4. Relieves pain
Jiao San Xian (*Jiao Mai Ya* + *Jiao Shang Zha* + *Jiao Shen Qu*)	焦三仙 (焦麦芽 +焦山楂 +焦神曲)	This is a term for three herbs in combination. Please refer to the individual herbs for English and Latin names.		1. Promotes digestion *Note: "Jiao" indicates that the herbs are fried continuously until charred. This helps to further enhance their effects in promoting digestion.*
Jie Geng	桔梗	*Radix Platycodi*	Platycodon Root	1. Promotes the dispersion of lung *qi* 2. Dispels phlegm 3. Soothes sore throat 4. Induces pus discharge of lung carbuncles
Jin Qian Cao	金钱草	*Herba Lysimachiae*	Longhairy Antenoron Herb	1. Removes dampness to treat jaundice 2. Promotes diuresis 3. Induces detoxification effect to reduce swelling

(*Continued*)

Table A.1. (*Continued*).

Name in *Pinyin*	Chinese Name	Latin Name	Common Name	Therapeutic Functions
Ju Hong	橘红	*Exocarpium Citri Grandis*	Pomelo Peel	1. Promotes the flow of *qi* to relieve *qi* stagnation in the abdomen 2. Removes dampness to resolve phlegm
Ju Ye	橘叶	*Citrus reticulata Blanco*	Tangerine Leaf	1. Disperses stagnation of liver *qi* 2. Disperses masses/ abnormal growth to reduce swelling
Lao Ling Ke	老菱壳	*Pedicellus et Pericarpium Trapae*	Water Calptrop Base and Peel	1. Induces astringency in the intestines to relieve diarrhoea 2. Stops bleeding 3. Detoxification effect
Lian Qiao	连翘	*Fructus Forsythiae*	Weeping Forsythia Capsule	1. Anti-inflammatory effect 2. Disperses masses/ abnormal growth to reduce swelling 3. Dispels exogenous wind-heat

(*Continued*)

Table A.1. (*Continued*).

Name in *Pinyin*	Chinese Name	Latin Name	Common Name	Therapeutic Functions
Liu Ji Nu	刘寄奴	*Herba Artemisiae Anomalae*	Diverse Wormwood Herb	1. Dissipates blood stasis to relieve pain 2. Stops bleeding which helps to promote healing of wounds 3. Strong effect on improving blood circulation to stimulate menstruation 4. Promotes digestion of residual food to relieve *qi* stagnation in the abdomen
Long Gu	龙骨	*Os Draconis/ Fossilia Ossis Mastodi*	Dragon's Bones, Fossilized	1. Calms the nerves and mind 2. Suppresses liver *yang* 3. Induces astringency in all body fluids *Note:* "Calcined" *means the herb has undergone the process of calcination, whereby ores/minerals are heated to bring about thermal decomposition. During the thermal treatment, calcium oxide is formed. This is to enhance its astringency effect on body fluids.*
Long Kui	龙葵	*Herba Solani Nigri*	Black Nightshade Herb	1. Anti-inflammatory effect 2. Promotes diuresis

(*Continued*)

Table A.1. (*Continued*).

Name in *Pinyin*	Chinese Name	Latin Name	Common Name	Therapeutic Functions
Lou Lü	漏芦	*Radix Rhapontici*	Uniflower Swisscentaury Root	1. Anti-inflammatory effect 2. Disperses masses to promote the healing of carbuncles 3. Stimulates menstruation 4. Promotes lactation 5. Removes blockage in collaterals and soothes the tendons to improve limb movements
Lu Jiao Jiao	鹿角胶	*Cervus nippon Temminck/ C. elaphus L.*	Deer Horn Glue	1. Tonifies the liver and kidney 2. Enriches the blood and essence
Lu Lu Tong	路路通	*Fructus Liquidambaris*	Beautiful Sweetgum Fruit	1. Removes wind-dampness in the collaterals to relieve rheumatic conditions, hence improving limb movements 2. Relieves oedema 3. Stimulates menstruation

(*Continued*)

Table A.1. (*Continued*).

Name in *Pinyin*	Chinese Name	Latin Name	Common Name	Therapeutic Functions
Luo Shi Teng	络石藤	*Caulis Trachelospermi*	Chinese Starjasmine Stem	1. Removes wind-dampness in the collaterals to relieve rheumatic conditions, hence improving limb movements 2. Cools the blood 3. Reduces swelling
Ma Dou Ling	马兜玲	*Fructus Aristolochiae*	Dutchmanspipe Fruit	1. Clears lung heat 2. Resolves phlegm 3. Anti-asthmatic effect and relieves cough 4. Clears intestine heat to treat piles
Ma Wei Lian	马尾连	*Radix et Rhizoma Thalictri*	Meadowrue Root and Rhizome	1. Removes damp-heat 2. Purges fire 3. Detoxification effect
Mai Ya	麦芽	*Fructus Hordei Germinatus*	Germinated Barley	1. Promotes digestion and strengthens the stomach functions 2. Relieves breast distension *Note: Parched* Mai Ya *indicates that it has undergone frying (炒); this enhances the effect of relieving breast distension.*

(*Continued*)

Table A.1. (*Continued*).

Name in *Pinyin*	Chinese Name	Latin Name	Common Name	Therapeutic Functions
Mao Zhua Cao	猫爪草	*Ranunculus ternatus Thunb*	Root of Catclaw Buttercup	1. Resolves phlegm to disperse masses/ abnormal growth 2. Induces detoxification effect to reduce swelling
Mu Li	牡蛎	*Concha Ostreae*	Oyster Shell	1. Calms the nerves and mind 2. Suppresses *yang* and strengthens *yin* 3. Softens and disperses masses/ abnormal growth *Note:* "Calcined" *means the herb has undergone the process by which ores/minerals are heated to bring about thermal decomposition. Calcium oxide is formed and this enhances the herb's astringency effect on body fluids.*
Mu Xiang	木香	*Radix Aucklandiae*	Costustoot	1. Promotes the flow of *qi* to relieve pain 2. Strengthens the spleen functions to promote digestion

(*Continued*)

Table A.1. (*Continued*).

Name in *Pinyin*	Chinese Name	Latin Name	Common Name	Therapeutic Functions
Nü Zhen Zi	女贞子	*Fructus Ligustri Lucidi*	Glossy Privet Fruit	1. Nourishes the liver and kidney 2. Promotes growth of black hair 3. Improves vision
Pi Pa Ye	枇杷叶	*Folium Eriobotryae*	Loquat Leaf	1. Clears lung heat to relieve cough 2. Relieves nausea and vomiting
Pu Gong Ying	蒲公英	*Herba Taraxaci*	Mongolian Dandelion Herb	1. Anti-inflammatory effect 2. Disperses masses/abnormal growth and reduces swelling 3. Promotes diuresis
Qian Cao	茜草	*Radix Rubiae*	India Madder Root	1. Stops bleeding by cooling the blood and removing blood stasis 2. Stimulates menstruation
Qian Hu	前胡	*Radix Peucedani*	Whiteflower Hogfennel Root/ Common Hogfennel Root	1. Resolves phlegm 2. Dispels exogenous wind-heat *Note: Frying the herb with honey helps to enhance the effects of nourishing and moistening the lung and resolving phlegm.*

(*Continued*)

Table A.1. (*Continued*).

Name in *Pinyin*	Chinese Name	Latin Name	Common Name	Therapeutic Functions
Qian Shi	芡实	*Semen Euryales*	Gordon Euryale Seed	1. Strengthens the kidney 2. Consolidates essence to treat involuntary seminal emission 3. Strengthens the spleen functions to relieve diarrhoea 4. Stops abnormal vaginal discharges (leucorrhoea) by removing dampness from the body
Qing Pi	青皮	*Pericarpium Citri Reticulatae Viride*	Green Tangerine Peel	1. Disperses stagnation of liver *qi* 2. Promotes digestion of food to relieve *qi* stagnation in the abdomen
Qu Mai	瞿麦	*Herba Dianthi*	Lilac Pink Herb	1. Promotes diuresis 2. Improves blood circulation and menstrual flow
Quan Xie	全蝎	*Scorpio*	Scorpion	1. Subdues endogenous wind to relieve convulsions 2. Counteracts toxins to disperse masses/abnormal growth 3. Clears blocked collaterals to relieve pain

(*Continued*)

Table A.1. (*Continued*).

Name in *Pinyin*	Chinese Name	Latin Name	Common Name	Therapeutic Functions
Ren Dong Teng	忍冬藤	*Caulis Lonicerae*	Japanese Honeysuckle Stem	1. Clears heat and expels wind 2. Clears blocked collaterals to relieve pain
Ren Shen	人参	*Panax Ginseng*	Ginseng	1. Invigorates *qi* 2. Tonifies the spleen and strengthens the lung 3. Promotes the production of body fluids 4. Calms the mind and improves alertness
Rou Dou Kou	肉豆蔻	*Terminalia Chebula*	Nutmeg	1. Arrests diarrhea 2. Arrests coughing 3. Clears voice
Rou Gui	肉桂	*Cortex Cinnamomi*	Cassia Bark	1. Reinforces *yang* 2. Dispels cold to relieve pain 3. Warms the meridians 4. Directs warm *yang* back to the kidney
San Qi	三七	*Panax Notoginseng*	—	1. Removes blood stasis to stop bleeding 2. Improves blood circulation 3. Relieves pain

(*Continued*)

Appendix 1

Table A.1. (*Continued*).

Name in *Pinyin*	Chinese Name	Latin Name	Common Name	Therapeutic Functions
Sang Bai Pi	桑白皮	*Cortex Mori*	White Mulberry Root-bark	1. Purges lung fire 2. Removes accumulated pleural fluids 3. Anti-asthmatic effect 4. Relieves oedema
Sang Zhi	桑枝	*Ramulus Mori*	Mulberry Twig	1. Removes wind-dampness in the collaterals to relieve rheumatic conditions, hence improving joint movements
Sha Yuan Zi	沙苑子	*Semen Astragali Complanati*	Flatstem Milkvetch Seed	1. Tonifies the kidney and consolidates the essence 2. Nourishes the liver 3. Improves vision
Shan Ci Gu	山慈菇	*Bulbus Iphigeniae Indicae*	Indian Iphigenia Bulb	1. Anti-inflammatory effect 2. Disperses masses to promote healing of carbuncles
Shan Dou Gen	山豆根	*Radix Sophorae Tonkinensis*	Vietnamese Sophora Root	1. Anti-inflammatory effect 2. Soothes sore throat 3. Reduces swelling

(*Continued*)

Table A.1.   (Continued).

Name in *Pinyin*	Chinese Name	Latin Name	Common Name	Therapeutic Functions
Shan Yao	山药	*Rhizoma Dioscoreae*	Common Yam Rhizome/ Winged Yam Rhizome/Wild Yam	1. Strengthens the spleen functions and nourishes the stomach 2. Promotes the production of body fluids 3. Strengthens the lung functions 4. Tonifies the kidney 5. Helps retention of *jing* (essence)
Shan Yu Rou	山萸肉	*Fructus Corni*	Asiatic Cornelian Cherry Fruit	1. Tonifies the liver and kidney 2. Astringent action on body fluids
Shan Zha	山楂	*Fructus Crataegi*	Hawthorn Fruit	1. Promotes digestion 2. Promotes the flow of *qi* 3. Dissipates blood stasis *Note: Parched* Shan Zha *indicates that the herb has undergone frying to enhance its effects of promoting digestion and resolving blood stasis.*
She Mei	蛇莓	*Herba Duchesneae Indicae*	Indian Mock Strawberry Herb	1. Removes heat in the blood 2. Reduces swelling 3. Detoxification effect

(Continued)

Table A.1. (*Continued*).

Name in *Pinyin*	Chinese Name	Latin Name	Common Name	Therapeutic Functions
Shen Qu	神曲	—	—	1. Promotes digestion and regulates the stomach functions *Note: Parched* Shen Qu *has undergone frying to enhance its effect of promoting digestion.*
Sheng Di Huang	生地黄	*Radix Rehmanniae*	Rehmannia Root	1. Removes heat in the blood 2. Nourishes *yin* 3. Promotes the production of body fluids
Sheng Jiang	生姜	*Zingiber officinale*	Ginger	1. Relieves the exterior syndrome and dispels cold 2. Warms the spleen and stomach to relieve nausea and vomiting 3. Warms the lung to relieve cough
Sheng Ma	升麻	*Rhizoma Cimicifugae*	Largetrifoliolious Bugbane Rhizome	1. Relieves the exterior syndrome 2. Promotes the breakout of measles 3. Anti-inflammatory effect 4. Uplifts *yang qi* to prevent the descent of *yang*

(*Continued*)

Table A.1. (*Continued*).

Name in *Pinyin*	Chinese Name	Latin Name	Common Name	Therapeutic Functions
Shi Hu	石斛	*Herba Dendrobii*	Dendrobium	1. Strengthens the stomach functions 2. Promotes the production of body fluids 3. Nourishes *yin* 4. Clears heat
Shi Jian Chuan	石见穿	*Herba Salviae Chinensis*	Chinese Sage Herb	1. Improves blood circulation and removes blood stasis 2. Removes damp-heat 3. Disperses masses/abnormal growth and reduces swelling
Shi Shang Bai	石上柏	*Herba Selaginellae Doederleinii*	Doederlein's Spikemoss Herb	1. Anti-inflammatory effect 2. Expels wind and dampness 3. Stops bleeding 4. Anti-cancer effect
Shi Wei	石韦	*Folium Pyrrosiae*	Pyrrosia Leaf	1. Promotes diuresis 2. Clears lung heat and relieves cough 3. Cools the blood to stop bleeding
Shou Wu Teng/Ye Jiao Teng	首乌藤/夜交藤	*Caulis Polygoni Multiflori*	Tuber Fleeceflower Stem	1. Nourishes the blood and calms the mind 2. Expels wind 3. Clears the blocked collaterals to relieve pain

(*Continued*)

Table A.1. (*Continued*).

Name in *Pinyin*	Chinese Name	Latin Name	Common Name	Therapeutic Functions
Shu Di Huang	熟地黄	*Radix Rehmanniae Preparata*	Rehmannia Root (prepared with wine)	1. Enriches the blood and nourishes *yin* 2. Supplements essence
Suan Zao Ren	酸枣仁	*Semen Ziziphi Spinosae*	Spina Date Seed	1. Nourishes the heart and strengthens the liver 2. Calms the nerves and mind 3. Astringent action to stop perspiration
Tai Zi Shen	太子参	*Radix Pseudostellariae*	Heterophylly False Starwort Root	1. Reinforces *qi* and strengthens the spleen 2. Promotes the production of body fluids to moisten the lung
Tao Ren	桃仁	*Semen Persicae*	Peach Seed	1. Improves blood circulation and removes blood stasis 2. Promotes bowel movement 3. Relieves cough 4. Anti-asthmatic effect
Teng Li Gen	藤梨根	*Radix Actinidiae Chinensis*	Actinidia Root	1. Anti-inflammatory effect 2. Removes dampness and expels wind 3. Promotes diuresis 4. Stops bleeding 5. Reduces swelling by inducing detoxification effect

(*Continued*)

Table A.1. (*Continued*).

Name in *Pinyin*	Chinese Name	Latin Name	Common Name	Therapeutic Functions
Tian Hua Fen	天花粉	*Radix Trichosanthis*	Mongolian Snakegourd Root	1. Clears heat and purges fire 2. Promotes the production of body fluids to quench thirst 3. Reduces swelling and induces pus discharge
Tian Kui Zi	天葵子	*Radix Semiaquilegiae*	Muskroot-like Semiaquilegia Root	1. Anti-inflammatory effect 2. Promotes diuresis 3. Disperses masses/ abnormal growth and reduces swelling
Tian Ma	天麻	*Rhizoma Gastrodiae*	Tall Gastrodia Tuber	1. Subdues endogenous wind to relieve convulsions 2. Suppresses liver *yang* 3. Expels wind 4. Clears blocked collaterals to relieve pain
Tian Men Dong/Tian Dong	天门冬/ 天冬	*Radix Asparagi*	Cochinchinese Asparagus Root	1. Nourishes *yin* to moisten dryness 2. Clears lung heat 3. Promotes the production of body fluids
Tu Bei Mu	土贝母	*Rhizoma Bolbostematis*	—	1. Disperses masses or abnormal growths 2. Reduces swelling 3. Detoxification effect

(*Continued*)

Name in *Pinyin*	Chinese Name	Latin Name	Common Name	Therapeutic Functions
Tu Fu Ling	土茯苓	*Rhizoma Smilacis Glabrae*	Glabrous Greenbrier Rhizome	1. Detoxification effect 2. Removes dampness 3. Promotes and improves joint movements
Tu Si Zi	菟丝子	*Semen Cuscutae*	South Dodder Seed/Chinese Dodder Seed	1. Tonifies the kidney and enriches essence 2. Nourishes the liver to improve vision 3. Relieves diarrhoea 4. Prevents miscarriage
Wang Bu Liu Xing/ Liu Xing Zi	王不留行/留行子	*Semen Vaccariae*	Cowherb Seed	1. Improves blood circulation to stimulate menstruation 2. Promotes lactation 3. Promotes the healing of breast carbuncles 4. Promotes diuresis
Wu Gong	蜈蚣	*Scolopendra*	Centipede	1. Subdues endogenous wind to relieve convulsions 2. Counteracts toxins to disperse masses/ abnormal growth 3. Clears blocked collaterals to relieve pain

(Continued)

Name in *Pinyin*	Chinese Name	Latin Name	Common Name	Therapeutic Functions
Wu Wei Zi	五味子	*Fructus Schisandrae*	Chinese Magnoliavine Fruit	1. Astringent action on body fluids 2. Strengthens *qi* 3. Promotes the production of body fluids 4. Tonifies the kidney 5. Calms the mind
Wu Yao	乌药	*Radix Linderae*	Combined Spicebush Root	1. Promotes the flow of *qi* to relieve pain 2. Warms the kidney and expels cold
Xia Ku Cao	夏枯草	*Spica Prunellae*	Common Selfheal Fruit-spike	1. Clears heat and purges fire 2. Improves vision 3. Disperses masses/abnormal growth to reduce swelling
Xue Li Guo	薛荔果	*Fructus Fici Pumilae*	Climbing Fig Fruit	1. Expels wind and dampness 2. Improves blood circulation to clear the blocked collaterals 3. Reduces swelling via detoxification effect
Ye Ju Hua	野菊花	*Flos Chrysanthemi Indici*	Wild Chrysanthemum Flower	1. Anti-inflammatory effect
Ye Pu Tao Gen	野葡萄根	*Radix Vitis Adstrictae*	Romanet Grape Root	1. Improves blood circulation 2. Promotes digestion to relieve abdomen distension

(Continued)

Table A.1. (*Continued*).

Name in *Pinyin*	Chinese Name	Latin Name	Common Name	Therapeutic Functions
Yi Yi Ren/ Yi Mi	薏苡仁	*Semen Coicis*	Coix Seed	1. Relieves oedema 2. Removes dampness from the spleen and collaterals to relieve diarrhoea and improve limb movements respectively 3. Strengthens the spleen functions 4. Clears heat and induces pus discharges from carbuncles
Yi Zhi Ren	益智仁	*Fructus Alpiniae Oxyphyllae*	Sharpleaf Galangal Fruit	1. Warms the kidney to consolidate essence, which helps to treat enuresis, polyuria and involuntary seminal emission 2. Warms the spleen to increase one's appetite and alleviate drooling (excessive saliva)
Yin Chen	茵陈	*Herba Artemisiae Scopariae*	Virgate Wormwood Herb/ Capillary Wormwood Herb	1. Removes dampness to treat jaundice 2. Induces detoxification effect to promote healing of wounds/ulcers

(*Continued*)

Table A.1.   (*Continued*).

Name in *Pinyin*	Chinese Name	Latin Name	Common Name	Therapeutic Functions
Yin Hua	银花	*Flos Lonicerae*	Honeysuckle Flower	1. Anti-inflammatory effect 2. Dispels exogenous wind-heat
Yu Jin	郁金	*Radix Curcumae*	Turmeric Root-tuber	1. Improves blood circulation to relieve pain 2. Promotes the flow of liver *qi* to relieve stagnation, which helps to treat depression 3. Clears heart heat and cools the blood 4. Improves the functions of the gallbladder which helps in the treatment of jaundice
Yu Xing Cao	鱼腥草	*Herba Houttuyniae*	Heartleaf Houttuynia Herb	1. Anti-inflammatory effect 2. Induces pus discharge which promotes the healing of carbuncles 3. Promotes diuresis
Yu Zhu	玉竹	*Rhizoma Polygonati Odorati*	Fragrant Solomonseal Rhizome	1. Nourishes *yin* to moisten dryness 2. Promotes the production of body fluids to quench thirst

(*Continued*)

Table A.1. (*Continued*).

Name in *Pinyin*	Chinese Name	Latin Name	Common Name	Therapeutic Functions
Yuan Hu/ Yan Hu Suo	元胡/延胡索	*Rhizoma Corydalis*	—	1. Improves blood circulation 2. Promote the flow of *qi* 3. Relieves pain
Yuan Zhi	远志	*Cortex et Radix Polygalae*	Thinleaf Milkwort Root-bark	1. Calms the mind and improves intelligence 2. Dispels phlegm 3. Reduces swelling and promotes the healing of carbuncles
Zao Jiao Ci	皂角刺	*Spina Gleditsiae*	Chinese Honeylocust Spine	1. Reduces swelling and induces pus discharge 2. Expels wind 3. Kills parasites
Zao Xiu	蚤休	*Paris Polyphylla*	Flea; Herba Violae	1. Clears heat and toxins 2. Reduces swelling and relieves pain 3. Cools liver
Ze Lan	泽兰	*Herba Lycopi*	Hirsute Shiny Bugleweed	1. Improves blood circulation to regulate menstruation 2. Removes blood stasis to aid in the healing of carbuncles 3. Relieves oedema

(*Continued*)

Table A.1. (*Continued*).

Name in *Pinyin*	Chinese Name	Latin Name	Common Name	Therapeutic Functions
Ze Xie	泽泻	*Rhizoma Alismatis*	Oriental Water Plantain Rhizome	1. Removes dampness to relieve oedema 2. Clears heat
Zhe Bei Mu	浙贝母	*Bulbus Fritillariae Thunbergii*	Thunberg Fritillary Bulb	1. Clears heat and resolves phlegm 2. Disperses masses/abnormal growth 3. Promotes the healing of carbuncles
Zhi Bai (Zhi Mu and Huang Bai)	知柏 (知母和 黄柏)	Please refer to each of the two herbs.		
Zhi Ke/Zhi Qiao	枳壳	*Fructus Aurantii*	Bitter Orange	1. Promotes the flow of *qi* to relieve stagnation in the chest and abdomen 2. Relieves abdomen distension
Zhi Mu	知母	*Rhizoma Anemarrhenae*	Common Anemarrhena Rhizome	1. Clears heat and purges fire 2. Promotes the production of body fluids to moisten dryness *Note: Frying Zhi Mu helps to reduce its effects of clearing heat and purging fire. This prevents damage to the spleen and stomach for individuals who have weak or impaired digestive systems.*

(*Continued*)

Table A.1. (*Continued*).

Name in *Pinyin*	Chinese Name	Latin Name	Common Name	Therapeutic Functions
Zhi Zi	栀子	*Fructus Gardeniae*	Cape Jasmine Fruit	1. Purges fire to ease irritability 2. Removes damp-heat 3. Cools the blood 4. Detoxification effect
Zhong Jie Feng	肿节风	*Herba Sarcandrae*	Glabrous Sarcandra Herb	1. Anti-inflammatory effect 2. Expels wind 3. Clears blocked collaterals to relieve pain 4. Improves blood circulation 5. Disperses masses/abnormal growth
Zhu Ru	竹茹	*Caulis Bambusae in Taeniam*	Bamboo Shavings	1. Clears heat and resolves phlegm 2. Relieves nausea and vomiting 3. Eases irritability
Zhu Yang Yang	猪殃殃	*Herba Galii Teneri*	Tender Catchweed Bedstraw Herb	1. Anti-inflammatory effect 2. Promotes diuresis 3. Reduces swelling
Zi Cao	紫草	*Radix Arnebiae/ Radix Lithospermi*	Sinkiang Arnebia Root/Redroot Gromwell Root	1. Removes heat in the blood 2. Improves blood circulation 3. Detoxification effect 4. Promotes the breakout of measles

(*Continued*)

Table A.1. (*Continued*).

Name in *Pinyin*	Chinese Name	Latin Name	Common Name	Therapeutic Functions
Zi He Che	紫河车	*Placenta Hominis*	Human Placenta	1. Tonifies the kidney and strengthens essence 2. Nourishes the blood and strengthens *qi*
Zi Wan/Zi Yuan	紫菀	*Radix Asteris*	Tatarian Aster Root	1. Nourishes the lung 2. Resolves phlegm and relieves cough

APPENDIX 2

COMMON FOODS WITH ANTI-CANCER EFFECTS*

The term "anti-cancer" (*kang ai* 抗癌) refers to the possibility of a herb inhibiting the growth of cancer cells; "preventing cancer" (*fang ai* 防癌) refers to the possibility of the herb contributing to the prevention of cancer. The evidence based on clinical trials for anti-cancer and cancer-preventing effects have not, in some instances, been firmly established or widely accepted, although in these instances there may be reasonable grounds based on preliminary or anecdotal evidence for believing that they have these effects. Table A.2 lists some common foods with anti-cancer effects.

---

* This list has been adapted from a table presented in Chinese from Professor Yu's 2008 book, *Yu Rencun Zhongxiyi Jiehe Zhongliu Xue* 郁仁存中西医结合肿瘤学, Peking Union Medical College Press, pp. 457–460.

Table A.2.   **Common Foods with Anti-Cancer Effects.**

Name of Food	Properties	TCM Functions	Findings from Modern Research Studies
Staple			
Soybean 大豆	—	1. Relieves stagnation in the upper abdomen, and promotes downward movement of *qi* 2. Reduces swelling 3. Detoxifies	High protein content of 36.6%, and rich in selenium. Incidence of malignancy occurring in gastric carcinoma dramatically decreases with long-term consumption of soybean by-products, such as tofu.
Wheat 小麦	Sweet in taste; cool in nature.	1. Nourishes the kidney and heart 2. Relieves dysphoria (irritability) 3. Quenches thirst	Non-specific boost in the immune system inhibits the development and progression of cancer. Polysaccharides in wheat bran have an inhibitory effect on the growth of sarcoma in mice.
Sesame 芝麻	Neutral-sweet in taste.	1. Nourishes the kidney 2. Invigorates the five organs: kidney, heart, liver, spleen and lung	Rich in protein. Antioxidant composition found in sesame is able to inhibit the development of tumours in animals.
Sweet potato 红薯	—	1. Nourishes *qi* in the body 2. Nourishes the spleen and kidney	Contains carotene, vitamin C, as well as eight other essential amino acids that the human body needs; has unique treatment effects for breast and colon cancer.

(Continued)

Table A.2.   (*Continued*).

Name of Food	Properties	TCM Functions	Findings from Modern Research Studies
Vegetables			
Sword bean 刀豆	Sweet in taste; warm in nature.	1. Dispels cold in the upper abdomen, and promotes downward movement of *qi* 2. Anti-emetic effect (prevents vomiting) 3. Promotes defecation 4. Nourishes the kidney	Sword bean contains haemagglutinin which converts lymphocytes into lymphoblasts. This in turn has an inhibitory effect on tumour development.
Fennel 小茴香	Acrid in taste; warm in nature.	1. Dispels cold in the kidney 2. Strengthens the stomach, and promotes *qi* circulation	Experimental studies have shown that fennel has an inhibitory effect on solid tumours, as well as the ability to increase white blood cell count.
Winter melon 冬瓜	Bland-sweet in taste; cool in nature.	1. Promotes elimination of heat through diuresis (urination) 2. Detoxifies 3. Dispels phlegm	Cucurbitacins that are contained in winter melon have an anti-cancer effect, preventing cancer from developing.
Cabbage 甘蓝 (包心菜、洋白菜)	Bland in taste; neutral in nature.	1. Aids in digestion through strengthening the spleen 2. Relieves stagnation in the chest 3. Relieves dysphoria (irritability) 4. Alleviates alcohol hangover, and promotes downward movement of *qi*	Cabbage contains indole–compounds, which inhibit the development of tumours in the animal gastrointestinal system. In addition, cabbage has an inhibitory effect on the development of human colon cancer.

(*Continued*)

Table A.2.   (*Continued*).

Name of Food	Properties	TCM Functions	Findings from Modern Research Studies
Kidney bean 四季豆	Sweet in taste; neutral in nature.	Strengthens the spleen and stomach	Plant haemagglutinin that is contained in kidney bean has an inhibitory effect on oesophageal cancer and hepatic cell line in humans, as well as an inhibitory effect on leukaemia development in mice; in addition, plant haemagglutinin is able to activate haemopoiesis in bone marrow, and interferon production in macrophages.
Tomato 西红柿	Sweet-sour in taste; cool in nature.	1. Eliminates heat, and quenches thirst 2. Nourishes *yin*, and eliminates heat in the blood 3. Anti-inflammatory effect 4. Promotes diuresis (urination)	It can prevent the occurrence of prostate cancer.
Bean sprout 豆芽	Sweet in taste; cool in nature.	1. Nourishes *yin*, and eliminates heat 2. Promotes diuresis (urination) 3. Detoxifies	There is an interferon-inducing element in bean sprout, which not only has an anti-viral function, but also an inhibitory effect on tumour development and progression.

(*Continued*)

Table A.2. (*Continued*).

Name of Food	Properties	TCM Functions	Findings from Modern Research Studies
Eggplant 茄子	Sweet in taste; cool in nature.	1. Improves blood circulation and removes stasis (blood clot) 2. Alleviates pain and swelling 3. Relieves stagnation in the intestines, and promotes diuresis (urination)	A certain non-toxic substance extracted from eggplant has a therapeutic effect on gastric, renal and cervical carcinoma.
Bitter gourd 苦瓜	Bitter in taste; cold in nature. Non-toxic.	1. Eliminates heat and improves vision 2. Detoxifies	Experimental studies have shown that bitter gourd is able to activate macrophages and boost the animal immune system. It is also shown that bitter gourd has an inhibitory effect on lymphoma.
Pumpkin 番瓜	Sweet in taste; warm in nature.	1. Strengthens the spleen and stomach 2. Nourishes *qi* 3. Anti-inflammatory effect 4. Alleviates pain 5. Detoxifies 6. Toxic effect on parasites	Pumpkin contains mannitol, a substance that promotes defecation. This reduces the toxins contained in the stools, which in turn reduces the harmful effects that these toxins may cause.

(*Continued*)

Table A.2. (*Continued*).

Name of Food	Properties	TCM Functions	Findings from Modern Research Studies
Hyacinth bean 扁豆	Sweet in taste; neutral in nature.	1. Nourishes the spleen, and alleviates diarrhoea 2. Eliminates heat and dampness	Plant haemagglutinin that is contained in hyacinth bean has the ability to boost the human immune system. It can also inhibit the growth of experimental tumours.
Carrot 胡萝卜	Acrid-sweet in taste; slightly warm in nature. Non-toxic.	1. Strengthens the spleen, and promotes circulation of *qi* 2. Strengthens the stomach and relieves stagnation in the chest	Carotene has the ability to prevent the occurrence of gastric, intestinal and nasopharyngeal carcinoma.
Cucumber 黄瓜	Sweet in taste; cool in nature.	1. Eliminates heat 2. Detoxifies 3. Promotes diuresis (urination) 4. Promotes secretion of body fluids	Cucumber is rich in cucurbitacins, which exhibit an inhibitory effect on the growth of experimental tumours. It has some preventive effects on the occurrence of oesophageal cancer.
Onion 葱	Acrid in taste; slightly warm in nature. Non-toxic.	1. Induces perspiration to relieve exterior syndrome 2. Dispels cold, and activates *yang* in body	It has the ability to reduce nitrite concentration in the stomach, thereby preventing the occurrence of gastric carcinoma. It also contains selenium, a trace element which exhibits a preventive effect on various carcinomas.

(*Continued*)

Table A.2. (*Continued*).

Name of Food	Properties	TCM Functions	Findings from Modern Research Studies
Fruits			
Red date 大枣	Sweet in taste; warm in nature.	1. Strengthens the spleen and stomach 2. Nourishes *qi* and blood	It contains a high concentration of vitamin C, which acts to prevent the occurrence of various tumours. It can also inhibit the carcinogenic effects brought about by guanidine nitrate in experimental tumours.
Hawthorn 山楂	Sweet-sour in taste; slightly warm in nature.	1. Aids in digestion through strengthening the stomach 2. Promotes blood circulation and removes stasis (blood clot)	Flavonoids that are contained in hawthorn are able to inhibit the active components of tumours; hawthorn decoction can also prolong the lives of tumour-bearing animals. Water extract from hawthorn has an inhibitory effect on ascites carcinoma and cervical carcinoma.
Fig 无花果	Sweet-sour in taste; neutral in nature.	1. Strengthens the spleen, and alleviates diarrhoea 2. Nourishes the lung, and eliminates heat in the pharynx	Fig has been shown to have an inhibitory effect on tumours in various animal models, such as transplanted sarcoma in rats, ascites carcinoma in mice and spontaneous mastocarcinoma in mice. It is able to activate an immune system cascade.

(*Continued*)

Table A.2. (*Continued*).

Name of Food	Properties	TCM Functions	Findings from Modern Research Studies
Plum 乌梅	Astringent-sour in taste; warm in nature.	1. Reduces swelling and solid masses 2. Promotes healing of sores 3. Toxic effect on parasites 4. Induces astringency in the lung and intestines	Water extract from plum has an inhibitory effect on various experimental tumours, such as sarcoma and ascites carcinoma in mice. Plum has also been shown to boost the immune system in humans.
Almond 杏仁	Bitter in taste; warm in nature. Contains low level of toxicity.	1. Relieves cough and asthma 2. Promotes defecation through lubrication of the intestines	Warm water extract of almond is able to inhibit human cervical carcinoma JTC-26. Active components in almond are also able to inhibit the growth of both sarcoma in rats and Ehrlich ascites carcinoma in mice.
Pomelo 柚子 (文旦)	Sweet-sour in taste; cold in nature.	1. Aids in digestion 2. Dispels phlegm 3. Strengthens the spleen 4. Promotes circulation of *qi*, and alleviates alcohol hangover	Pomelo extract has exhibited inhibitory rates of 70–90% on human cervical carcinoma. Naringin in grapefruits can effectively protect mice from radiation injury, thereby suggesting the possibility of pomelo being used as a medicine in chemotherapy, against radiation injury.

(*Continued*)

Table A.2. (*Continued*).

Name of Food	Properties	TCM Functions	Findings from Modern Research Studies
Banana 香蕉	Sweet in taste; cold in nature.	1. Eliminates heat and promotes diuresis (urination) 2. Promotes defecation 3. Reduces blood pressure	Banana extract has been shown to exhibit a drastic inhibitory effect on the active components of carcinogens, such as aflatoxin and benzopyrene. Bananas are rich in trace element magnesium, which can prevent cancer from occurring.
Strawberry 草莓	Sweet-sour in taste; cool in nature.	1. Nourishes the lung, and promotes secretion of body fluids 2. Strengthens the spleen 3. Alleviates alcohol hangover	Strawberry is rich in vitamin C, which has an inhibitory effect on the production of potent carcinogens, nitrosamines. Strawberry amines contained in strawberries are effective in the treatment of leukaemia and aplastic anaemia.
Water chestnut 菱角	Sweet in taste; neutral in nature.	1. Eliminates heat and promotes secretion of body fluids 2. Relieves dysphoria (irritability) and cough 3. Strengthens the spleen, and nourishes *qi*	Water chestnuts have been used by common folks in the treatment of oesophageal carcinoma, gastric carcinoma, cervical carcinoma and mastocarcinoma. The fruit of the water chestnut has an inhibitory effect on ascitic hepatoma AH-13.

(*Continued*)

Table A.2. (*Continued*).

Name of Food	Properties	TCM Functions	Findings from Modern Research Studies
Kiwifruit 猕猴桃	Sweet-sour in taste; cool in nature.	1. Eliminates heat and promotes diuresis (urination) 2. Promotes secretion of body fluids, and relieves dryness in the body	Kiwifruit can block the carcinogenic effects of nitroso compounds. It can also improve the appetite of patients suffering from tumours, as well as maintain the blood count of patients undergoing chemotherapy.
Edible Fungi			
Black fungus 云耳 (黑木耳)	Sweet in taste; neutral in nature.	1. Strengthens the spleen, and nourishes *qi* 2. Nourishes the lung 3. Invigorates the brain 4. Nourishes the blood	Polysaccharides contained in black fungus have an inhibitory effect on sarcoma S_{180} in animals. It also has a therapeutic effect on cervical carcinoma and vaginal carcinoma.
Oyster mushroom 平菇	Sweet in taste; slightly warm in nature.	1. Strengthens the spleen, and relieves dampness 2. Relaxes muscles and joints by promoting circulation of blood	Polysaccharides contained in oyster mushrooms have an inhibitory rate of 75.3% on sarcoma S_{180} in mice. Constant intake of oyster mushrooms can increase metabolism, and regulate autonomic functions in humans.

(*Continued*)

Table A.2. (*Continued*).

Name of Food	Properties	TCM Functions	Findings from Modern Research Studies
Mushroom 香菇	Sweet in taste; neutral in nature.	1. Strengthens the spleen and kidney 2. Nourishes *qi*, and stimulates appetite	Polysaccharides contained in mushrooms have a good inhibitory effect on leukaemia, as well as on other tumours, such as oesophageal, gastric, colorectal, lung and hepatic carcinoma. It is currently being used clinically, in the form of intravenous treatment.
White fungus 银耳 (白木耳)	Bland-sweet in taste; neutral in nature.	1. Nourishes *yin* and the lung 2. Strengthens the stomach, and promotes secretion of body fluids 3. Strengthens the kidney	Polysaccharides contained in white fungus have been found to increase the tolerance level to radiation and chemical drugs, as well as enhance the immune system in experimental animals. It is able to inhibit tumour S_{180} through these mechanisms.

(*Continued*)

Table A.2. (*Continued*).

Name of Food	Properties	TCM Functions	Findings from Modern Research Studies
Hedgehog fungus 猴头菌	Sweet in taste; neutral in nature.	1. Strengthens the spleen, and nourishes *qi* 2. Invigorates the five organs: kidney, lung, heart, liver and spleen	Polysaccharides and the polypeptide component contained in hedgehog fungus exhibit an inhibitory effect on gastric carcinoma and tumour S_{180} in mice. It has been shown to inhibit the synthesis of DNA and RNA in cancer cells, *in vitro*. It is also able to enhance the immune system in humans.
Meat, Poultry, Seafood			
Clam 文蛤	Salty in taste; neutral in nature.	1. Eliminates heat in the lung 2. Dispels phlegm 3. Disperses solid masses	Extracts of clam liver have been shown to prolong the lives of animals with leukaemia. Extracts of sterigmatocystin clams exhibit an inhibitory effect on tumour S_{180}, Ehrlich ascites carcinoma and leukaemia L_{1210} in animal models.
Tortoise 乌龟	Sweet-sour in taste; warm in nature.	1. Nourishes the kidney and liver 2. Disperses wind syndrome and eliminates dampness syndrome	It is able to boost the immune system, and has an inhibitory effect on tumours in animal models, such as tumour S_{180} and ascitic hepatoma in mice.

(Continued)

Table A.2. (*Continued*).

Name of Food	Properties	TCM Functions	Findings from Modern Research Studies
Turtle 甲鱼 (团鱼、水鱼)	Sweet in taste; neutral in nature.	1. Strengthens the liver and kidney 2. Nourishes *qi* and blood	The rich collagen molecule content of turtles can improve the nutritional status and metabolism rate, thereby alleviating cachexia in cancer patients. The shell of turtles has an inhibitory effect on experimental tumours such as hepatic carcinoma and gastric carcinoma.
Chicken 鸡肉	Sweet in taste; warm in nature.	1. Strengthens the stomach and spleen 2. Nourishes *qi* 3. Invigorates essence of the kidney	Some studies have claimed that using 100°C boiling water to cook chicken for 2 minutes is able to kill the cancer cells that may be contained in the chicken.
Oyster 牡蛎	Salty-sweet in taste; neutral in nature.	1. Nourishes *yin* and blood 2. Invigorates the heart 3. Tranquilizes the mind	Water extract of oyster has a direct inhibitory effect on tumours in voles. Oyster contains elements that have a cytotoxic effect on experimental tumours.
Hairtail 带鱼	Sweet in taste; warm in nature.	1. Warms the stomach 2. Provides nourishment for deficiency syndromes 3. Moisturizes the skin	6-Thioguanine is an anti-cancer compound that can be found in the scales of hairtails, which can be effectively used for the treatment of leukaemia and other malignant tumours.

(*Continued*)

Table A.2. (*Continued*).

Name of Food	Properties	TCM Functions	Findings from Modern Research Studies
Sea cucumber 海参	Sweet in taste; warm in nature.	1. Strengthens the kidney, and invigorates essence of the kidney 2. Boosts male vitality 3. Dispels phlegm	Holothurin contained in sea cucumber is able to inhibit the growth of some experimental tumours, such as tumour S_{180} and Ehrlich ascites carcinoma.
Earthworm 蚯蚓	Salty in taste; cold in nature.	1. Eliminates heat by relieving stagnation of *qi* in the liver 2. Alleviates asthma by promoting circulation of blood	It has an inhibitory effect on colorectal carcinoma, hepatic carcinoma and cervical carcinoma–26 in humans.
Crab 螃蟹	Salty in taste; cold in nature.	Crab meat: 1. Eliminates heat, and disperses solid masses 2. Nourishes *yin* and promotes circulation of blood 3. Promotes healing of external injuries Crab shell: 1. Eliminates heat 2. Detoxifies 3. Removes stasis (blood clot) and disperses solid masses	Crab shell has been shown to be effective in the treatment of mastocarcinoma.

(*Continued*)

Table A.2.   (*Continued*).

Name of Food	Properties	TCM Functions	Findings from Modern Research Studies
Shark 鲨鱼	Sweet in taste; neutral in nature.	1. Strengthens the spleen 2. Nourishes *qi* 3. Invigorates blood	Shark is rich in vitamin A, which can help in the prevention of cancer. Active components extracted from shark's fin can prevent the occurrences of experimental tumours in animals.
Others			
Pollen 花粉	Sweet in taste; neutral in nature.	Reduces body weight, and prolongs life span on long-term usage	In a survey carried out in France, it was found that only 1 out of 1000 apiarists died from cancer. Animal experiments have shown that pollen has the ability to inhibit the growth of cancer cells.
Honey 蜂蜜	Sweet in taste; neutral in nature.	1. Invigorates *qi*, and relieves dryness in the body 2. Nourishes the lung, and relieves cough 3. Detoxifies 4. Alleviates pain	Ether-soluble compounds contained in honey have an inhibitory effect on experimental tumours, such as leukaemia, lymphoma, mastocarcinoma and Ehrlich ascites carcinoma.

(*Continued*)

Table A.2.   (*Continued*).

Name of Food	Properties	TCM Functions	Findings from Modern Research Studies
Yoghurt 酸奶	—	—	Yoghurt has been shown to have an inhibitory effect on some transplanted experimental tumours.
Royal jelly 蜂王浆	Sweet in taste; slightly warm in nature.	Has strong nourishing effect	Royal jelly has an inhibitory effect on experimental tumours, such as leukaemia, lymphoma, mastocarcinoma and Ehrlich ascites carcinoma. It can also prolong the lives of mice suffering from cancer.
Vinegar 醋	Bitter-sour in taste; warm in nature.	1. Removes stasis (blood clot), and stops bleeding 2. Detoxifies 3. Toxic effects on parasites	It can inhibit the carcinogenic effect of aflatoxin.

INDEX